ADHD Diagnosis: Beyond Averages

Sanobar

First Printing, 2024

Table of Contents

Review of Literature

This book aimed to investigate the diagnostic utility of intraindividual variability (IIV) in determining Attention Deficit/Hyperactivity Disorder (ADHD) status in a group of children ages 6 to 13 years old. The following review of the literature begins with a discussion of IIV in a typically developing population, the relationship between IIV and attention abilities, ways of defining and statistically estimating IIV, and current understandings of the neural correlates of IIV. Following this, there will be a discussion of IIV in clinical populations including neurodegenerative and neurodevelopmental disorders. This will then lead into a discussion of ADHD, the primary focus of this book, including ADHD's diagnosis, etiology, treatment, behavioural and neural correlates, relationship with IIV, and relevant theories.

Intraindividual Variability

In statistics, the variability of scores refers to the dispersion or spread of those scores. Previously, any variability in an individual's scores over a short period of time was thought to solely be due to error or noise. However, while some level of variation in performance, such as an individual's performance on a single measure, can be indeed due to error such as fatigue or practice effects, it is now well established in the literature that there is a degree of that variability that is clinically meaningful because it is no longer random, but is instead characteristic of an individual's performance (Nesselroade, 1991).

Hultsch, MacDonald, and Dixon, (2002) defined three types of variability; diversity, dispersion, and inconsistency. Diversity represents variability seen *between* persons on a single task and testing occasion while both dispersion and inconsistency represent variability seen *within* person. Dispersion represents the variability in an individual's scores across multiple measures, such as differences in standard scores across measures of memory, attention, and problem-solving. Inconsistency represents the variability in performance of a single person, on a single task, across multiple occasions spanning the short-term (multiple trials on the same day or over days) or long-term (multiple testing occasions over weeks, months, or longer periods). This study focuses on short-term inconsistency, specifically multiple trials of a task within a single test administration.

The time-scale on which inconsistency is measured is also worth noting given that inconsistency in the short-term is thought to represent unique cognitive processes when compared to inconsistency in the long term (Li, Huxhold, & Schmiedek, 2004; MacDonald, Li, & Bäckman, 2009). Specifically, inconsistency in the long-term (e.g., over months or years) has been thought to be representative of slow and relatively permanent changes that may be the result of maturation over time and/or learning (Li et al., 2004; MacDonald, Li, et al., 2009). On the other hand, inconsistency in the short term, which can be measured in day-to-day variability in performance, may at times be unrelated to cognitive abilities, and instead be dependent on the individual's current state (e.g., stress; Sliwinski, Smyth, Hofer, & Stawski, 2006). Inconsistency on an even smaller time scale (e.g., trial-to-trial) is thought to be a behavioural indicator of the integrity of the brain and its processes including attention and executive control (e.g., Albaugh et al., 2016; Bielak, Hultsch, Strauss, MacDonald, & Hunter, 2010; Kelly, Uddin, Biswal, Castellanos, & Milham, 2008; Li et al., 2004; MacDonald, Nyberg, & Bäckman, 2006; MacDonald & Stawski, 2015). Relatedly, trial-to-trial inconsistency has been shown to reliably distinguish atypically developing individuals (e.g., ADHD,

Autism Spectrum Disorder, traumatic brain injury, and dementia) from healthy controls, and thus is considered to be of clinical relevance as a useful behavioral marker for underlying neural pathology (MacDonald et al., 2006). In the current study and from here on, the term intraindividual variability (IIV) is used to refer to inconsistency in the short-term; that is, within-person trial-to-trial variability on a single task (e.g., Hultsch et al., 2002).

Estimating IIV.

While there are various statistical approaches to estimating IIV as defined here, many methods rely on response times (RT; measured in milliseconds) from multiple trials of a single task, which is often computerised to facilitate accurate RT recordings and has limited demand on language/reading ability due to visual stimuli (such as an object or single letter), simple instructions and limited response requirements, such as pressing a single button (Hultsch, Strauss, Hunter, & MacDonald, 2008). One of the frequently used and simpler methods of estimating IIV is intraindividual standard deviation (ISD), also known as RT standard deviation (RTSD), which is the standard deviation calculated using one individual's RT on multiple trials (Kofler et al., 2013). This method has been criticized because it fails to account for the influence of that individual's mean RT on their variability, as the two are often highly correlated (Hultsch et al., 2008). In fact, Wagenmakers and Brown (2007) noted a linear correlation between RT mean and SD such that larger means tended to have larger SDs. Researchers have attempted to overcome this limitation by using the intraindividual coefficient of variability (ICV) which is calculated by dividing ISD by mean RT, supposedly decoupling IIV from mean RT (Hultsch et al., 2008). Taking this even further is the residual ISD (rISD) approach to estimating IIV where systematic within-person variations, such as fatigue or practice effects, are partialled out in a linear regression analysis before estimating IIV, resulting in a 'purer' measure (Hultsch et al., 2008). The statistical methods that underlie these approaches (ISD, ICV, and rISD), however, rely on the assumption that the RTs are normally distributed which, particularly for children with ADHD, may not be the case (Leth-Steensen, Elbaz, & Douglas, 2000). Specifically, Leth-Steensen, Elbaz, and Douglas, (2000) found that the RT distribution of children with ADHD differed from age-matched controls such that for ADHD, the RT distribution was characterised by a large positive skew indicating a greater proportion of slower responses (See also Hervey et al., 2006). As a result, the previously mentioned methods of estimating IIV may not be appropriate for this population since the RT mean and ISD of the ADHD group may be inflated due to the longer responses that contributed to the large positive skew (Hervey et al., 2006; Leth-Steensen et al., 2000).

One method that accounts for a skewed RT distribution while estimating IIV, and that is likely better able to characterise IIV in children with ADHD, is the ex-Gaussian approach (e.g., Castellanos, Sonuga-Barke, Milham, & Tannock, 2006; Hervey et al., 2006; Leth-Steensen, Elbaz, & Douglas, 2000). This method assumes that there are two components to the RT distribution; RTs that are normally distributed (Gaussian), and those that are exponentially distributed (ex). As a result, it disentangles these two components into μ and σ, the mean and standard deviation of the normal component respectively, and τ, the combined mean and standard deviation of the exponential component (i.e., the abnormally slower responses). Overall, τ is thought to represent IIV, while μ and σ are thought to represent a general slowing of RT and deficits in motor timing or a measure of dispersion, respectively (Leth-Steensen et al., 2000; Vaurio, Simmonds, & Mostofsky, 2009). Research using the ex-Gaussian approach with children with ADHD has shown that the increase in IIV in this population appears largely due to elevations in τ, while μ and σ are often comparable to controls or differences are smaller in magnitude compared to τ (e.g., Buzy, Medoff, & Schweitzer, 2009; Hervey et al., 2006; Karalunas & Huang-Pollock, 2013; Leth-Steensen et al., 2000). This finding suggests that it is the abnormally slow responses that may be driving increased variability in this population. In other words, children with ADHD are not necessarily slower in response times on average, but they are more variable in their responding due to a greater number of slow responses (e.g., Buzy, Medoff, & Schweitzer, 2009; Epstein et al., 2011; Henríquez-Henríquez et al., 2015; Leth-Steensen, Elbaz, & Douglas, 2000; Lin, Hwang-Gu, & Gau, 2015). This finding would otherwise be lost if earlier mentioned estimates of IIV such as ISD, ICV or rISD were used to calculate IIV within this population. For this reason, the current study will use the ex-Gaussian approach to estimate IIV based on its strong support in the ADHD literature (e.g., Henríquez-Henríquez et al., 2015; Hervey et al., 2006; Lee et al., 2015; Leth-Steensen et al., 2000; Schmiedek, Oberauer, Wilhelm, Süß, & Wittmann, 2007; Tamm et al., 2012).

IIV over the typically developing lifespan.

With respect to typical development, IIV over the lifespan has been noted to take on a U-shaped curve (Dykiert, Der, Starr, & Deary, 2012; Williams, Hultsch, Strauss, Hunter, & Tannock, 2005). Specifically, using ISD, Williams and colleagues (2005) found that IIV is high in childhood (under 12 years), begins to decrease during adolescence (ages 13-17 years) and young adulthood (ages 18-29 years), and then begins to increase again with greater age throughout middle adulthood (ages 30-44 years), older adulthood (ages 45-59 years) and late adulthood (over 59 years). Differences in IIV patterns are thought to be related to changes occurring in the brain such that high IIV in young children is associated with the developmental immaturity of their neural connections and lower IIV in adolescence to adulthood is reflective of white matter maturation in the brain (i.e. increased efficiency; Tamnes, Fjell, Westlye, Ostby, & Walhovd, 2012). The final increase in IIV from middle adulthood to older adulthood is associated with cognitive decline and normative degeneration in the brain (Bielak, Cherbuin, Bunce, & Anstey, 2014; Bielak et al., 2010; Haynes, Bauermeister, & Bunce, 2017; MacDonald et al., 2006) including reduced white matter integrity (Jackson, Balota, Duchek, & Head, 2012).

Williams, Hultsch, Strauss, Hunter, and Tannock (2005) concluded, based on their analyses of the RT distribution for different age groups, that high IIV in younger individuals is likely due to both general information processing deficits and specific deficits such as lapses of attention (likely due to immaturity of the still developing brain rather than pathological causes), compared to older individuals where lapses of attention appeared to be the main contributor to IIV. Interestingly, Brennan, Bruderer, Liu-Ambrose, Handy, and Enns (2017) were able to replicate previous research, using an ecologically valid task (e.g., entering a room and visually searching for items), suggesting that attention abilities as measured using a visual search task also presented with a U-shaped function (similar to that of IIV) such that search time and errors were high in both childhood and older adulthood, but lower in young and middle adulthood (See also

Hommel, Li, & Li, 2004). This finding suggests an overlap between IIV and attention development over the lifespan.

Neural correlates of IIV in a healthy population.

A growing body of literature has focused on determining the neural correlates of IIV in an attempt to shed light on the underlying neural processes associated with IIV, though this area has been dominated by research in typical adulthood and aging, with few studies focused on typically developing children. Studies using structural magnetic resonance imaging (MRI) in a healthy adult population have noted an association with IIV and white matter integrity of the brain, including reduced volume (Walhovd & Fjell, 2007), increased hyperintensities reflective of microlesions (Bunce et al., 2010, 2007), as well as non-specific white matter changes as revealed through diffusion tensor imaging (DTI; Moy et al., 2011). The reduction of white matter volume with aging is related to reduced myelination of axons that allow for efficient communication between neurons, and may also be a contributing factor to the increased IIV seen in older adults (Walhovd & Fjell, 2007). Bunce and colleagues (2007) reported an association between white matter hyperintensities (indicating lesions) in the frontal lobes and increased IIV in an older population (ages 60-64), though this association may be stronger in women during middle adulthood (ages 44-48; Bunce et al., 2010). They hypothesized that the relationship between the frontal lobe hyperintensities and IIV likely reflects the impact of pathology in the brain that may result in attention lapses or reduced executive control that contribute to increased IIV (Bunce et al., 2007).

In terms of the functional neural correlates of IIV in a typically developing population, IIV has been related to activity in regions involved in attention processes including frontal and prefrontal cortex (Bellgrove, Hester, & Garavan, 2004; Simmonds et al., 2007), inferior parietal cortex (MacDonald, Nyberg, Sandblom, Fischer, & Bäckman, 2008), anterior cingulate cortex (ACC; Johnson et al., 2015), the default-mode network (DMN; Kelly et al., 2008), the P-300 response which is considered an index of attention allocation and executive control (Ramchurn, de Fockert, Mason, Darling, & Bunce, 2014), and diminished dopamine binding (D2 receptor) in extrastriatal regions (ACC, orbitofrontal cortex, and hippocampus; MacDonald, Cervenka, Farde, Nyberg, & Bäckman, 2009). Specifically, low IIV on an inhibitory task using functional MRI (fMRI) has been associated with the rostral pre-supplementary motor area (pre-SMA) in children (Simmonds et al., 2007), while high IIV has been associated with increased activity in frontal and pre-frontal regions for both children and adults (Bellgrove et al., 2004; Simmonds et al., 2007). These findings have been discussed as likely representing the relationship between high IIV and suboptimal state regulation (including motivation and attention to task) such that the individual's suboptimal state resulted in less automatic activation of the pre-SMA during task response and they instead needed to recruit frontal regions (Bellgrove et al., 2004; Simmonds et al., 2007). IIV is also related to increased competition between brain regions active during on-task behaviour and the DMN (a network of brain regions that are active at rest and suppressed during goal-directed behaviour; Kelly et al., 2008). That is, increased IIV is related to a reduced ability to suppress the DMN which has been found to be associated with lapses of attention (Weissman, Roberts, Visscher, & Woldorff, 2006). Additionally, research by Adleman and colleagues (2016) found that the relationship between IIV and trial-by-trial changes to the blood oxygenated level dependent (BOLD) response in fMRI (what the authors refer to as the RT-BOLD relationship) strengthens with age over childhood into adulthood. Specifically, Adleman et al. (2016) report an age-dependent variation in the RT-BOLD relationship in various regions of the brain associated with attention which they hypothesize is related to developmental changes to attention processes over childhood and into adulthood.

Another noteworthy area of research related to IIV is neural variability. Specifically, neural variability (within subject variability of brain signals) is noted to be negatively correlated with behavioural variability (i.e., IIV); that is, low levels of neural variability are related to high levels of IIV and vice versa (McIntosh, Kovacevic, & Itier, 2008). Neural variability is typically measured using neuroimaging techniques with a focus on moment-to-moment fluctuations in brain signals (See Garrett et al. (2013) for a review). While increased IIV is associated with poorer performance on cognitive tasks, neural variability appears to be beneficial such that high neural variability is associated with improved efficiency in cognitive processing (Dinstein, Heeger, & Behrmann, 2015; Garrett et al., 2013; Renart & Machens, 2014). This high neural variability is hypothesized to represent increased flexibility of neural networks or a state that is ready to respond and thus results in more stable behavioural output (Dinstein et al., 2015; Garrett et al., 2013; McIntosh et al., 2008; Renart & Machens, 2014). Compared to the U-shaped function of IIV across the lifespan, Garrett and colleagues (2013) proposed an inverted U-shape function of neural variability based on their review of various studies, such that neural variability is low in childhood and increases with age into adulthood (possibly reflecting a limited repertoire of possible responses during which IIV is high and then begins to decrease), after which neural variability begins to decline with increasing age into older adulthood (while IIV is low and begins to increase with age).

Overall IIV in a typically developing population is related to various structural and functional regions in the brain that appear to be involved in attention and executive control processes. However, these are not necessarily mutually exclusive but may instead interact in some way, though additional research is needed in this area. Research regarding IIV in a typically developing population has provided a yard stick of sorts to determine whether measured IIV in an individual is within the expected range. When IIV shows differences beyond the optimal/expected level (e.g., increased IIV), then this may be an indicator of underlying damage or pathology in the brain. Indeed, increased IIV is noted in clinical populations that commonly experience attention difficulties including traumatic brain injury (e.g., Stuss, Murphy, Binns, & Alexander, 2003), dementia (e.g., Haynes et al., 2017), Fetal Alcohol Spectrum Disorder (FASD; e.g., Ali, Kerns, Mulligan, Olson, & Astley, 2017), Autism Spectrum Disorder (ASD; e.g., Adamo et al., 2014), and ADHD (e.g., Kofler et al., 2013).

IIV in Clinical Populations

Attention deficits have been noted as a common cognitive outcome following traumatic brain injury (Beaulieu-Bonneau, Fortier-Brochu, Ivers, & Morin, 2017; Sinclair, Ponsford, Rajaratnam, & Anderson, 2013), and while findings of greater IIV in concussed individuals have been inconclusive (Cole, Gregory, Arrieux, & Haran, 2017; Karr, Garcia-Barrera, & Areshenkoff, 2014; Sosnoff, Broglio, Hillman, & Ferrara, 2007), there is evidence to suggest that IIV is elevated in more severe injuries (Hill, Rohling, Boettcher, & Meyers, 2013; Sinclair et al., 2013; Stuss et al., 2003). Specifically, using a choice-RT task with four levels of increasing complexity, Stuss and colleagues (2003) demonstrated that patients with frontal lobe lesions were more variable compared to those with non-frontal lesions and non-injured controls, suggesting that increased IIV in that population may be due to impairments in the top-down control of attention.

In an older adult population, atypically high IIV, as well as impairments in attention, is present in neurodegenerative diseases such as dementia, Parkinson's and mild cognitive impairment (Bharath et al., 2017; Burton, Strauss, Hultsch, Moll, & Hunter, 2006; Haynes et al., 2017; Hultsch, MacDonald, Hunter, Levy-Bencheton, & Strauss, 2000; Jackson et al., 2012; Murtha, Cismaru, Waechter, & Chertkow, 2002; Tang et al., 2016). In fact, a recent review noted atypical IIV often precedes, and is predictive of, cognitive decline and even death in an older population (Haynes et al., 2017). Additionally, high IIV has been linked to compromised white matter integrity (including the frontal lobes) in older adults such that lower white matter volume is related to higher IIV (Jackson et al., 2012), which the authors suggest is associated with failures in executive and attentional control mechanisms.

Atypical IIV is also noted in neurodevelopmental disorders such as ASD and FASD; however, due to the severity of attention impairment reported in these diagnoses, ASD and FASD are often co-morbid with ADHD (Ali et al., 2017; Burd, 2016; Gargaro, Rinehart, Bradshaw, Tonge, & Sheppard, 2011; Karalunas, Geurts, Konrad, Bender, & Nigg, 2014). As a result, the high incidence of these co-morbidities makes it difficult to tease apart whether the levels of IIV noted are specific to ASD or FASD, or if they are more related to broad attention impairment and comorbid ADHD (Ali et al., 2017; Karalunas et al., 2014). In fact, Adamo et al. (2014) found that children with ASD plus

ADHD symptoms had levels of IIV comparable to children with ADHD alone, while those with ASD who had no ADHD symptoms were indistinguishable from controls (See also Biscaldi et al. (2016)). These findings suggest that IIV may represent a unique underlying pathology associated with ADHD, or more specifically, impairments of attention. A review of IIV research specific to ADHD follows.

Attention Deficit/Hyperactivity Disorder

ADHD is a neurodevelopmental disorder seen in approximately 5% of the childhood population and is characterised by functional impairments in attention and/or hyperactivity-impulsivity (American Psychiatric Association, 2013). In children, ADHD is twice as likely to be diagnosed in boys and although onset is in childhood, ADHD symptoms can persist into adulthood with an adult prevalence of approximately 2.5% (American Psychiatric Association, 2013). In addition to difficulty with attention and/or hyperactivity/impulsivity, individuals with ADHD often experience secondary problems over their lifespan including difficulties with mood, learning, substance abuse, health-related quality of life, and overall life satisfaction (Elia, Ambrosini, & Berrettini, 2008; Y. Lee et al., 2016; Lensing, Zeiner, Sandvik, & Opjordsmoen, 2015; Schei, Jozefiak, Nøvik, Lydersen, & Indredavik, 2016; Tarver, Daley, & Sayal, 2014).

Diagnosis.

In North America, ADHD is diagnosed based on symptoms outlined in the Diagnostic and Statistical Manual of Mental Disorders, Fifth Edition (DSM-5; American Psychiatric Association (2013)). There are three presentations of ADHD that can be diagnosed: (1) the predominantly inattentive presentation, where the child meets a minimum of 6 out of 9 inattention symptoms, (2) the predominantly hyperactive/impulsive presentation, where the child meets a minimum of 6 out of 9 hyperactive/impulsive symptoms, and (3) the combined presentation where the child meets a minimum of 6 out of 9 symptoms on both the inattentive and hyperactive/impulsive domains. These symptoms must have been present before 12 years of age, seen in multiple settings, interfere with daily functioning, and not be due to another disorder (See Appendix C). The International Classification of Diseases (ICD-10; WHO (2004)) is used to diagnose ADHD (also known as Hyperkinetic Disorder) in Europe, and other regions outside of North America, and outlines similar criteria to the DSM-5. However, although similar diagnostic criteria are used, the ICD-10 does not specify subtypes and it is considered to have 'stricter' requirements such as requiring at least six out of nine inattention, three out of five hyperactivity, and one out of four impulsivity symptoms for diagnosis of the disorder. The higher prevalence rates of ADHD in North America compared to Europe is thus likely due to the stricter criteria required by ICD-10 as well as the fact that pervasive developmental disorders such as Autism cannot be co-morbid with ADHD under ICD-10, but this is possible under DSM-5 (Doernberg & Hollander, 2016; Parens & Johnston, 2009). Overall, the difference between the DSM-5 and ICD-10 criteria for diagnosis is relatively small (Tripp, Luk, Schaughency, & Singh, 1999) and the upcoming review of literature regarding IIV in ADHD does not distinguish whether ADHD was diagnosed using DSM or ICD criteria.

The current guidelines for the diagnosis of ADHD are largely based on informant ratings (e.g., parents and teachers) documenting the child's functional impairment in multiple settings (e.g., American Academy of Pediatrics, 2011); however, this approach has limitations (Ford-Jones, 2015; Parens & Johnston, 2009). In a recent review of the literature, Ford-Jones (2015) reported that children who are younger than their same-grade peers (e.g., born closer to the start of the school year) are more likely to receive a diagnosis of ADHD, suggesting a failure on the part of informants to account for the developmental immaturity of younger children in the classroom. This is concerning when stimulant medication is used as treatment without a clear understanding of potential side-effects, especially in cases where the target behaviours may have improved naturally with age (Ford-Jones, 2015). Additionally, they reported that boys are more likely to be diagnosed with ADHD than girls, due to boys having increased behavioural (hyperactive/impulsive) symptoms and therefore being more readily identified by teachers (Ford-Jones, 2015). This under-diagnosis of girls means that those who would benefit from intervention are not identified, which may compromise their academic achievement (Ford-Jones, 2015) and lead to other secondary effects such as lower quality of life, which has been shown to be significantly reduced following early diagnosis and intervention (Coghill, Banaschewski, Soutullo, Cottingham, & Zuddas, 2017; Sonuga-Barke, Koerting, Smith, McCann, & Thompson, 2011).

Relatedly, due to the reliance on informant ratings based on observation, Parens and Johnston (2009) report that children often fall into the 'zone of ambiguity', such that there is debate on whether their symptoms are severe enough to warrant a diagnosis. This means that the decision to provide the diagnosis falls on the physician/psychologist who may be responding to parental/teacher distress (Parens & Johnston, 2009). The authors also noted that in some cases children are diagnosed when they meet the symptom list criteria with insufficient information on level of impairment, and those with subthreshold symptoms but high levels of impairment may not receive a diagnosis or appropriate intervention (Parens & Johnston, 2009).

Another difficulty with diagnosing ADHD is the DSM-5's final diagnostic criteria which requires that symptoms are not due to another cause such as mood disorder, learning disorders, or brain injury, which may be difficult to establish given the rates of co-morbidity between ADHD and these diagnoses (American Psychiatric Association, 2013; Tarver et al., 2014). Additionally, these rule-out diagnoses also lead to similar difficulties with attention though for different reasons, which essentially results in ADHD being somewhat a diagnosis of exclusion, though its diagnosis is rarely conducted as such when using DSM-5 guidelines. Instead, although not best-practice, diagnosis is often reliant on one or two brief rating scales which tend to only have modest agreement between caregivers and teachers (Ali, Macoun, Bedir, & MacDonald, 2019; Lavigne, Gouze, Hopkins, & Bryant, 2016; Narad et al., 2015; Sims & Lonigan, 2012). Sims and Lonigan (2012) suggested that the discrepancy between raters may be due to genuine differences in behaviours observed (i.e., behaviours differ between settings) or differences in the salience of those behaviours in different settings (i.e., some behaviours may be more disruptive in a classroom environment compared to the home.)

Due to the problematic reliance on subjective rating scales outlined above, researchers have attempted to identify objective measures of diagnosing ADHD, including the use of cognitive testing. A meta-analysis of continuous performance tests (CPT) in children with ADHD found large effect sizes for commission and omission errors, as well as IIV using SDRT (Huang-Pollock, Karalunas, Tam, & Moore, 2012). However, a recent systematic review on the utility of CPTs in aiding diagnosis of ADHD,

Hall et al. (2016) found that while CPTs were a good way of objectively assessing attention and impulsivity in children, results were inconclusive regarding their ability to improve accuracy of an ADHD clinical diagnosis. Specifically, they noted that the test of variables of attention (TOVA) measure of 'variability' (ISD) was helpful in distinguishing children with ADHD from those without, but the addition of other TOVA variables did not improve predictive power, and the overall TOVA score was unable to distinguish children with ADHD from those with subthreshold symptoms (Hall et al., 2016). Additionally, the low ecological validity of CPT tasks, and the artificial environment (i.e., quiet, highly structured, with limited distractions) in which it is completed may result in false negatives (Sims & Lonigan, 2012).

As implied by the above review of CPTs, one possible solution in the search for a reliable cognitive marker may be IIV (Hall et al., 2016). However, based on previously mentioned shortcomings to using SDRT and ISD as a measure of IIV in an ADHD population, the ex-Gaussian approach may prove to be a valuable alternative in determining the utility of CPTs (Leth-Steensen et al., 2000). Therefore, the question remains whether IIV using ex-Gaussian analysis can aid in the ADHD diagnostic process by helping to distinguish children with ADHD from those whose attention difficulties are not so severe as to warrant a diagnosis.

Etiology of ADHD.

There is no clear consensus on the cause of ADHD, and it is likely that the cause varies between individuals, which may include genetic factors, environmental factors, or some combination of the two (Tarver et al., 2014). Based on family and twin studies, ADHD is considered to be a heritable disorder however, no single gene has been implicated (Faraone et al., 2005; Thapar, Cooper, Eyre, & Langley, 2013). In their review, Thapar and colleagues (2013) noted the candidate genes consistently associated with ADHD include dopaminergic genes (DAT1, DRD4, and DRD5), serotonergic genes (5HTT and HTR1B), a neuron specific protein (SNAP-25), and the COMT genotype which regulates dopamine concentrations. The main environmental risk factors implicated with ADHD includes maternal smoking (e.g., Froehlich et al., 2009; Knopik et al., 2016; Silva, Colvin, Hagemann, & Bower, 2014), maternal stress (e.g., Grizenko, Fortier, Gaudreau-Simard, Jolicoeur, & Joober, 2015), low birth weight (e.g., Pereira, Da Mata, Figueiredo, de Andrade, & Pereira, 2017), lead exposure (e.g., Froehlich et al., 2009; Goodlad, Marcus, & Fulton, 2013; Nigg, 2010; Thapar et al., 2013), dietary factors (e.g., Tarver et al., 2014; Thapar et al., 2013), and the family environment including early neglect (e.g., Maguire et al., 2015), parenting styles (e.g., Haack, Villodas, Mcburnett, Hinshaw, & Pfiffner, 2016; Muñoz-Silva, Lago-Urbano, & Sanchez-Garcia, 2017), and socioeconomic status (e.g., Rowland et al., 2017; Russell, Ford, Williams, & Russell, 2016).

Neural correlates in ADHD.

The prefrontal cortex has consistently been implicated in both structural and functional studies of ADHD (e.g., Bush, 2011; Durston, Van Belle, & De Zeeuw, 2011; Friedman & Rapoport, 2015; Krain & Castellanos, 2006; Liston, Cohen, Teslovich, Levenson, & Casey, 2011). Relatedly, the frontostriatal network, which includes reciprocal connections between the prefrontal cortex, thalamus, and striatum, has also received much attention in ADHD (Cubillo, Halari, Smith, Taylor, & Rubia, 2012; Durston et al., 2011; Rubia, 2011; Rubia et al., 2011; Schneider et al., 2010; Schweren et al., 2016; van Ewijk, Heslenfeld, Zwiers, Buitelaar, & Oosterlaan, 2012) with some studies suggesting improvements in these circuits following treatment with stimulant medication (Rubia et al., 2011; Schweren et al., 2016). Durston and colleagues (2011) reviewed three circuits implicated in ADHD including the dorsal frontostriatal circuit involved in cognitive control (e.g., response inhibition, switching and planning), the orbitofrontal-striatal circuit involved in reward and motivation, and the fronto-cerebellar circuit involved in timing. The authors suggest that deficits in any of these three circuits can lead to symptoms of ADHD and propose the use of neurobiological subtypes based on these circuits, though additional research is needed in this area (Durston et al., 2011).

While there is much evidence to support the involvement of the prefrontal cortex and its connections with other neural regions in ADHD, it is not the only implicated region (Castellanos & Proal, 2012; Chen et al., 2016; Friedman & Rapoport, 2015; Krain & Castellanos, 2006). Recent reviews on the structural neural findings in ADHD highlight reduced total brain volumes, where the four lobes (frontal, temporal, occipital, and parietal) are equally affected, in children with ADHD compared to controls (Friedman & Rapoport, 2015; Krain & Castellanos, 2006). In addition to the prefrontal cortex, reduced volumes have been noted in the basal ganglia, corpus callosum, cerebellum, and parieto-temporal regions (Friedman & Rapoport, 2015; Krain & Castellanos, 2006) which have been reported to be correlated with increased symptom severity as well as poorer performance on neuropsychological measures (for a review see Krain & Castellanos, 2006). Additionally, a systematic review and meta-analysis of DTI studies using tract-based spatial statistics (TBSS) reported abnormalities in WM tracts connecting the left and right hemisphere (corpus callosum splenium) and posterior brain pathways, including the occipital and temporal lobes, which the authors suggest might be related to symptoms of inattention, distractibility, and visual dysfunctions (Chen et al., 2016).

In an attempt to expand focus beyond the frontostriatal circuit, Castellanos and Proal (2012) propose that ADHD may be best conceptualised in a more inclusive brain model that consists of deficits in the dorsal attention, visual, motor, and default-mode networks, including connections between and within networks. Relatedly, a recent study regarding functional connectivity in the brains of children with ADHD compared to controls, reported that children with ADHD showed increased local connectivity in attention related networks compared to controls suggesting an immaturity of the connections, such that mature connections would be more global in nature (Marcos-Vidal et al., 2018). These authors also noted a correlation between the local connectivity patterns in somatosensory regions and symptom severity for both children with and without ADHD (Marcos-Vidal et al., 2018).

Regarding neural variability, recall that in typically developing individuals, high neural variability has been associated with better cognitive outcomes such that the brain is considered to be continuously in a state that is ready to respond (Garrett et al., 2013; McIntosh et al., 2008). On the other hand, neural variability research using EEG in individuals with ADHD has found abnormally high levels of variability in brain signals compared to controls (Gonen-Yaacovi et al., 2016; McLoughlin, Palmer, Rijsdijk, & Makeig, 2014; Saville et al., 2015). Specifically, Gonen-Yaacovi and colleagues (2016) noted that abnormally large levels of neural variability were recorded in ADHD, and it was continuous rather than specific to sensory or cognitive functions, as reported by others (McLoughlin et al., 2014; Saville et al., 2015), supporting the whole-brain approach to understanding ADHD.

Overall, while neural correlate research in individuals with ADHD was previously dominated by questions regarding the involvement of the prefrontal cortex and frontostriatal circuits, recent work has highlighted the need to apply a whole-brain approach when conceptualising the neural underpinnings of ADHD. Structural and functional research has implicated various regions involving all four lobes as well as connections within and between hemispheres, and specific networks including, but not limited to, the visual, motor, attention and default-mode networks (e.g., Castellanos & Proal, 2012; Chen et al., 2016; Friedman & Rapoport, 2015; Krain & Castellanos, 2006). Finally, research has also implicated unusual activity at the neuronal level in ADHD (e.g., Gonen-Yaacovi et al., 2016). These neural findings will later be discussed within the context of IIV in ADHD.

Treatments of ADHD.

Treatments for ADHD focus on the reduction of symptoms and functional impairment and include pharmacological and non-pharmacological interventions (detailed reviews: Findling, 2008; Sonuga-Barke et al., 2013; Vaughan, March, & Kratochvil, 2012). Pharmacological interventions include stimulant medications, such as methylphenidate (e.g., Ritalin) and amphetamine (e.g., Adderall) which are typically the first line of treatment, or non-stimulants such as atomoxetine (e.g., Strattera) or guanfacine (e.g., Intuniv; Thapar & Cooper, 2016). Both stimulants and non-stimulants are efficacious in their treatment of core ADHD symptoms (Hanwella, Senanayake, & de Silva, 2011; Hazell et al., 2011) as well as improving quality of life and reducing functional impairments (Coghill et al., 2017). Non-pharmacological interventions typically include changes to the individual's diet (Nigg, Lewis, Edinger, & Falk, 2012; Pelsser, Frankena, Toorman, & Pereira, 2017; Sonuga-Barke et al., 2013), and psychological interventions including behavioural management and cognitive training (Evans et al., 2014). The efficacy of these non-pharmacological interventions also remain inconclusive (Evans et al., 2014; Sonuga-Barke et al., 2013).

Regardless of treatment choice, early intervention has been discussed as having the potential for positive outcomes, both regarding core symptoms of ADHD as well as secondary outcomes such as academic achievement and quality of life (Coghill et al., 2017; Halperin, Bédard, & Curchack-Lichtin, 2012; Sonuga-Barke & Halperin, 2010). Specifically, Sonuga-Barke and Halperin (2010) rationalize that establishing a way to identify children in need of intervention before their symptoms appear, possibly through developmental processes that may mediate ADHD, would be more beneficial than the current method of diagnosing based on symptoms and then intervening. They discuss that early intervention (starting in pre-school years) may alter developmental trajectories through brain plasticity, as well as before behaviours become habituated and before complications with secondary aspects appear, thus improving overall outcome, though such an approach is yet to be empirically assessed (Sonuga-Barke & Halperin, 2010). For early intervention to be beneficial, the individual needs to first be identified at an earlier stage, rather than awaiting severe symptom presentation. In other words, a sensitive objective marker (such as increased IIV if empirically established as such), needs to be identified.

IIV and ADHD

While there is no specific cognitive profile of children with ADHD, deficits are commonly noted on aspects of executive function (including working memory), attention, and increased IIV (Kuntsi, McLoughlin, & Asherson, 2006; Thapar & Cooper, 2016). IIV findings have been one of the more consistent outcomes noted such that atypical levels of IIV have been reported in both children/adolescents and adults with ADHD (Kofler et al., 2013; Kuntsi & Klein, 2011; Tamm et al., 2012), and it appears to be independent of gender (Uebel et al., 2010). In a meta-analysis of 319 studies conducted between 1972 and 2011, Kofler and colleagues (2013) reported that children with ADHD had higher levels of IIV compared to typically developing controls even when ADHD presentation and motor processing speed was accounted for. They also noted that while those with ADHD were more variable, they were not necessarily slower on average in their responding, with their increased IIV being driven by a subset of abnormally slow responses (based on ex-Gaussian analysis; Kofler et al., 2013; Hervey et al., 2006).

Due to the consistency of IIV findings in ADHD, IIV has been proposed as an endophenotype of the disorder by multiple researchers using a variety of IIV estimates (e.g., ex-Gaussian and ISD; Bidwell, Willcutt, DeFries, & Pennington, 2007; Castellanos & Tannock, 2002; Frazier-Wood et al., 2012; Henríquez-Henríquez et al., 2015; Lin et al., 2015; Nigg, Blaskey, Stawicki, & Sachek, 2004; Pinto, Asherson, Ilott, Cheung, & Kuntsi, 2016). To be considered an endophenotype, a trait must be heritable and reliable in its connection with known genetic causes of a disease. Specifically, studies with children with ADHD, their unaffected siblings, other family members, and controls have shown somewhat of a stepwise relation with IIV independent of IQ and other cognitive abilities, implicating its heritability and utility as an endophenotype (Bidwell et al., 2007; Henríquez-Henríquez et al., 2015; Nigg et al., 2004; Thissen et al., 2014). Relatedly, genetic research using twins has noted an association with IIV and specific genes implicated in ADHD including IIV mediating the relationship between a serotonin receptor gene and inattention, as well as its association with dopaminergic genes (Cho et al., 2008; Frazier-Wood et al., 2012; Kebir & Joober, 2011; Kebir, Tabbane, Sengupta, & Joober, 2009; Pinto et al., 2016). Finally, the stimulant medication Methylphenidate has been found to improve IIV in children and adults with ADHD (Bédard et al., 2015; Epstein, Brinkman, et al., 2011; Kofler et al., 2013; Ni et al., 2016; Spencer et al., 2009), while the impact of non-stimulant medications for ADHD (e.g., Atomoxetine) is variable. The inconclusive findings regarding non-stimulant medication and IIV may be due to the indicator of IIV used, such that use of non-stimulant medication was found to decrease IIV when the ex-Gaussian parameter τ was used (Ni et al., 2016), but not when ISD was used (Bédard et al., 2015). As previously mentioned, the method of estimating IIV in ADHD may be an important consideration in that the ex-Gaussian approach accounts for the large skew typically seen in the ADHD response curve while the ISD method may not fully capture that feature, and possibly account for mixed results across various studies (Leth-Steensen et al., 2000).

Greater levels of IIV have been noted in ADHD compared to controls regardless of ADHD presentation; however, findings are varied with respect to whether the levels of IIV noted between ADHD presentations is equivalent (Kofler et al., 2013; Tamm et al., 2012). Specifically, Kofler and colleagues (2013) noted in their meta-analysis that while IIV between the presentations was similar, the ADHD-combined and hyperactive/impulsive presentation were somewhat more variable compared to the inattentive presentation; therefore, it is unclear whether IIV is more closely related to behavioural expressions of inattention or hyperactivity/impulsivity, or both. IIV was also comparable when clinical control groups were used leading authors to question whether IIV is likely a broad marker of attention pathology rather than specific to ADHD (Kofler et al., 2013). This is in contrast to the conclusions of other studies (Henríquez-Henríquez et al., 2015; Leth-Steensen et al., 2000) though these authors did not employ a clinical control group.

Behavioural correlates of IIV in ADHD.

Regarding its behavioural correlates in ADHD, IIV has been linked to subjective measures of inattention (Antonini, Narad, Langberg, & Epstein, 2013; Gomez-Guerrero et al., 2011) and hyperactivity (Gomez-Guerrero et al., 2011). Specifically, Antonini and colleagues (2013) found that IIV was positively related to observations of off-task behaviour which they associate with behavioural inattention. Additionally, research has found that IIV significantly explained variance in parent and teacher ratings of ADHD symptoms including attention, hyperactivity, inhibition, emotional control, behavioural regulation, and monitoring (Ali, Macoun, Bedir, et al., 2019; Gomez-Guerrero et al., 2011).

IIV has also been linked to objective performance on tasks of attention, specifically increased distractibility on an oculomotor task (Adams et al., 2011), and performance on motor (Klotz, Johnson, Wu, Isaacs, & Gilbert, 2012), working memory (Kofler et al., 2014), and reading tasks (Tamm et al., 2014). The impact of IIV on self-paced academic tasks such as reading is an area of ongoing investigation. Studies have found a relationship between IIV (based on inter-item pause variability on a self-paced naming task e.g., Rapid Automatized Naming) and reading fluency (Ryan et al., 2017) and reading comprehension (J. J. Li et al., 2009), which the authors suggest is due to lapses of attention driven by inefficient top-down response control, including poor effort allocation and processing speed. Interestingly, Tamm and colleagues (2014) have noted a unique association between IIV (as measured by ISD on a stop signal task, i.e., an externally paced task) and word reading, which secondarily affected reading fluency and reading comprehension. The authors did not find a relationship between processing speed and reading ability, and they hypothesized that IIV may be reflective of information processing and executive control failures which impact reading ability (Tamm et al., 2014). The implications for these findings suggest that IIV can have an impact on academic achievement in this population (Borella, Chicherio, Re, Sensini, & Cornoldi, 2011; J. J. Li et al., 2009; Ryan et al., 2017; Tamm et al., 2014).

Neural correlates of IIV in ADHD.

Similar to research in a typically developing population, focus is increasingly being placed on understanding the neural correlates of IIV in ADHD and if, or how, they differ from findings noted in the general population. As with a healthy population, IIV has been found to be related to white matter abnormalities in an ADHD group (Hong et al., 2015; Lin et al., 2014; Mahone et al., 2011; Rossi et al., 2015; Wolfers et al., 2015). Specifically, various measures of IIV have been found to be related to reduced integrity of white matter tracts including those connecting frontal regions involved with attention (Lin et al., 2014; Rossi et al., 2015; Wolfers et al., 2015) as well as white matter volume in the supplementary motor cortex (Mahone et al., 2011). Interestingly, Mahone and colleagues (2011) conducted separate analyses for boys and girls with ADHD and in addition to both groups having reduced white and grey matter volume in the supplementary motor cortex, boys independently had reduced white matter in the left medial prefrontal cortex which the authors hypothesized accounts for reduced executive control of behaviour in boys. Girls with ADHD on the other hand, had reduced grey matter volume in the left lateral premotor cortex, an area they found to be related to IIV, which suggests that inattention and increased IIV may be due to poor maintenance of response control in girls (Mahone et al., 2011). Additional structural findings specific to ADHD include higher IIV being related to lower grey matter volumes in the ventromedial prefrontal cortex which plays a role in the DMN (Albaugh et al., 2016), and reduced total and grey matter brain volume (Greven et al., 2015).

Regarding the functional neural correlates of IIV and ADHD, some parallels exist with research using a typically developing population including association with reduced P3 amplitudes using event-related potentials (Cheung et al., 2017), reduced activity in the DMN, specifically the ventromedial PFC (Fassbender et al., 2009) and reduced BOLD activation in ACC (Rubia, Smith, Brammer, & Taylor, 2007). Interestingly, Cheung et al (2017) used two conditions, baseline and fast-rate of stimuli presentation, and they found that while the ADHD group was able to reduce their IIV from the baseline to the fast-rate condition, in association with an increase in P3 amplitude, the ADHD group overall had higher IIV which was in general associated with attenuated P3 amplitudes, suggesting difficulties with attentional resource allocation. Saville and colleagues (2015) however, in their electroencephalography (EEG) study concluded that group difference in IIV between their ADHD group and controls was less related to attention, and more related to response processes, though they did not fully rule out the role of attention in IIV broadly.

fMRI research thus far seems to suggest that increased IIV in children with ADHD may be related to their reliance on compensatory motor regions, possibly due to delayed maturity of frontal, attention related, regions (Rubia et al., 2007; Suskauer et al., 2008). Research by Rubia and colleagues (2007) noted that medication naïve children with ADHD in general showed less activation in areas that mediate attention allocation including the superior and middle temporal lobes. Regarding IIV, they noted that high IIV in the ADHD group was related to activity in the basal ganglia and thalamus, as well as reduced activity in the anterior cingulate cortex which may be due to this group having to rely on compensatory regions due to a delay in maturation of attention networks (based on reduced superior and middle temporal lobe activation; Rubia et al., 2007). On the other hand, high IIV in controls was related to activation in the superior temporal lobe which implicates a relationship between IIV and attention allocation at least in the control group (Rubia et al., 2007). Similarly, research by Suskauer and colleagues (2008) noted that children with ADHD and high IIV showed increased activation in motor areas, specifically the pre-SMA, while those with lower IIV had increased activation in frontal regions. This is notably in contrast to findings in a typical population where increased frontal activation was associated with high IIV (Simmonds et al., 2007). These findings suggest that children with ADHD were able to overcome this variability by imposing greater cognitive control during the task through activation of pre-frontal regions (Suskauer et al., 2008). In other words, it may be that children with ADHD who were able to exert greater attentional control to complete the task, showed lower variability.

Unfortunately, the relationship between IIV and ratings of attention problems were not discussed in these studies, leading to the question of whether high IIV is related to significantly greater clinical manifestations of inattention. Of note, these authors used ICV as a measure of IIV rather than the ex-Gaussian model of estimating IIV.

As mentioned in the earlier section on neural correlates in ADHD, atypically high levels of neural variability have been noted in ADHD compared to a typically developing population (Gonen-Yaacovi et al., 2016). Interestingly, these authors did not find a correlation between neural variability and IIV while a negative relationship has been noted in typically developing individuals (McIntosh et al., 2008). Nevertheless, additional research is needed to understand the relationship, if any, between neural variability and IIV in an ADHD population as it is clear that relationships similar to a typical population are unlikely to exist given the number of differences noted here on neural activity in individuals with ADHD compared to a typically developing population.

Overall, research on neural correlates of IIV in individuals with ADHD suggest a relationship between IIV and aspects of attention allocation. These include reduced white matter integrity and volume in regions associated with attention and motor responses, increased competition between the DMN and task-specific regions, reduced attention resource allocation via executive control mechanisms, and possibly a delayed development of regions associated with attention. There is also significant overlap between these above mentioned regions specific to IIV in ADHD, and broad neural findings in ADHD independent of IIV research, which provides support for the argument that these deficits may not be mutually exclusive and instead variably contribute to symptoms of ADHD including deficits of attention and elevated levels of IIV (Castellanos & Proal, 2012).

Theories of ADHD and how they account for IIV.

There is no single accepted theory that explains IIV in ADHD, though the predominant theories are not necessarily mutually exclusive. In other words, current IIV theories may have similar interpretations about what IIV in ADHD represents (e.g., failures of attention), but different explanations for why it exists in those with ADHD (e.g., top-down versus bottom-up control), or explain different aspects of IIV (e.g., fast versus slow end of the response curve). These explanations range from deficits in information processing in neural regions, to inefficient energy allocation, to task-specific factors. The widely discussed theories are reviewed below.

Theories that link IIV in ADHD with attention include the response time distribution approach of Leth-Steensen, Elbaz, and Douglas (2000) who, in their discussion of response times and τ using the ex-Gaussian approach, suggest that high IIV in boys with ADHD compared to same age peers is not a result of general slowing of responses, but of occasional excessively longer response times which produces a larger tail in the response curve (i.e., τ). They suggest these longer response times may be due to poor allocation of effort which may lead to attention lapses during information processing (Leth-Steensen et al., 2000). They also compared the ADHD group with younger controls and found no difference in τ which they hypothesized represented a delay in development of attention abilities in the ADHD group (Leth-Steensen et al., 2000). The relationship with attention failures and increased IIV was later reproduced by Hervey et al. (2006) using a larger sample of children on a CPT task. Contributing to this hypothesis that IIV is a result of attention difficulties is the finding that stimulant medication reduces IIV in children with ADHD independent of the medication's effect on motor speed (Bédard et al., 2015; Epstein, Brinkman, et al., 2011; Kofler et al., 2013; Ni et al., 2016; Spencer et al., 2009). The relationship between IIV and attention is less direct in Barkley's (1997) behavioural inhibition theory of ADHD, which posits that behavioural inhibition is the core deficit in children with ADHD. This core deficit results in executive dysfunction including working memory and self-regulation, which in turn impact sustained attention and motor control (Barkley, 1997). This implies that IIV may be due to poor sustained attention secondary to deficits in behavioural inhibition (Barkley, 1997; Kofler et al., 2013).

Based on the results from neuroimaging studies, theories have been proposed regarding the relationship between IIV, attention abilities and processes in the brain, of which the default-mode hypothesis and the executive control hypothesis are often discussed (Bellgrove et al., 2004; Castellanos, Kelly, & Milham, 2009; Fassbender et al., 2009; Huang-Pollock et al., 2012; Sonuga-Barke & Castellanos, 2007; Weissman et al., 2006). The default-mode hypothesis of ADHD views increased IIV as resulting from attention lapses due to a failure to deactivate the DMN during a task (Castellanos et al., 2009; Fassbender et al., 2009; Sonuga-Barke & Castellanos, 2007; Weissman et al., 2006). These lapses theoretically are attributable to the increased competition between the DMN and task-specific processes which results in longer RTs and ultimately increased IIV (Sonuga-Barke & Castellanos, 2007). Alternatively, increased RTs that contribute to higher IIV have been discussed as due to failures in executive control processes (reduced efficiency of top-down attentional control; Bellgrove et al., 2004) or slower information processing (Huang-Pollock et al., 2012; Karalunas, Nigg, & Huang-Pollock, 2012).

Some authors have investigated whether IIV is affected by specific task factors such as inter-stimulus intervals or slowing following an error (Epstein et al., 2010; Hervey et al., 2006). Specifically, Epstein et al. (2010) conducted a 'microanalysis' of task events (e.g., omission and commission errors), and reported that children with ADHD had slower RTs both before and after an omission error. The slowing before the omission error may be due to reduced engagement and task monitoring resulting in the omission error, and the continued slowing after the error is likely the continuation of these processes, that is, continued inattention (Epstein et al., 2010). RT slowing was also noted to follow a commission error and as discussed by the authors, this implies that increased IIV may be due to task-related factors, such that the RT slowing following the error contributed to IIV. However, when these trials (RT related to omission and commission errors) were removed, IIV in children with ADHD remained higher than controls, which suggest that IIV may be influenced by both task-related factors and ongoing fluctuation of attention unrelated to task parameters (Epstein et al., 2010).

Hervey and colleagues (2006), in addition to supporting the relationship between IIV and inattention, noted that IIV increased as the inter-stimulus interval increased (i.e., IIV increased as the time between stimulus presentation increased). The authors suggest that along with lapses of attention, this positive correlation may be due to a change in cognitive energy levels or, alternatively, the longer inter-stimulus intervals meant more chances for distraction (Hervey et al., 2006). They link this with the cognitive energetic model of ADHD (Russell et al., 2006; Sergeant, 2005) which suggests that an optimal energy level needs to be present to meet task demands and that this process is dysfunctional in children with ADHD (Sergeant, 2005). Russell and collegues (2006) further suggest that increased IIV in children with ADHD is a result of inefficiency of neural signalling due to this reduced energy availability. Specifically, they suggest that astrocytes in the central nervous system (CNS), which provide energy to neurons and support myelination (and thus efficient neurotransmission), are unable to provide a sufficient energy supply to rapidly firing neurons which leads to inconsistent performance (Russell et al., 2006). This inconsistent performance may be related to deficiencies in motor organisation which Sergeant (2005) includes as a mechanism of attention in the cognitive energetic model. Furthermore, the use of rewards during task performance also improves IIV which may be related to effort or energetic factors (Tye et al., 2016), and this improvement is similar both in children with ADHD and controls (Epstein, Langberg, et al., 2011). Overall, although task-related factors appear to play some role in IIV, they do not fully account for the higher levels of IIV noted in ADHD groups, suggesting that underlying attention abilities may, at least in part, account for this ongoing increase in IIV.

Relatedly, using fast fourier transform (FFT) analysis, Johnson and colleagues (2007) investigated IIV in children with ADHD stratified by impaired and unimpaired performance on a Sustained Attention Response Task (SART). They reported that the SART-impaired ADHD group showed higher IIV in the slow and fast frequency bands which they hypothesized to be related to low arousal and deficits in sustained attention respectively (Johnson et al., 2007). The SART-unimpaired group, however, did not show such a relationship which led the authors to conclude that children with ADHD may have different neural abnormalities that result in similar symptomology (i.e., same symptoms but different underlying neural contributors). Additionally, this finding suggests that IIV may be closely tied to attention abilities rather than the ADHD diagnosis which, as previously mentioned, is based on subjective informant reports.

In summary, most theories of ADHD attribute IIV to momentary lapses of attention that lengthen response times, though they differ in their explanations of what are the underlying physiological cause of these lapses. While it appears that task-related factors play some role in IIV, they do not fully account for the increase in IIV seen in ADHD, suggesting that underlying attention abilities also play a role. Whether the cause of these lapses is due to deficiencies in energy allocation, failure to suppress the default mode network, inefficiencies in top-down control of attention resources or some combination of these factors, it remains the case that attention may play a key role in increased IIV in ADHD. The theory that most closely aligns with the current study, is the response time distribution theory of Leth-Steensen at al., (2000) who noted that high IIV in ADHD is due to an increased amount of slow response times likely due to lapses of attention during the task. IIV is estimated using the ex-Gaussian parameter τ, which targets these particularly slow responses. As a result, based on the previously reviewed literature, which suggests that a relationship exists between IIV and attention, including research indicating increased IIV in clinical groups experiencing symptoms of inattention and the relationship between IIV and neural regions associated with attention, there is support for investigating IIV and its relationship with attention abilities on a continuum as well as its utility in diagnosing ADHD.

Objectives and Hypotheses

Research of IIV in children thus far has compared children with ADHD to typically developing children, or other clinical groups (e.g., ASD). Here, the relationship between IIV and attention will be investigated with respect to a continuum of attention abilities using the ex-Gaussian approach; that is, determining whether IIV shows a predictive linear relationship with levels of attention impairment. The current study aims to use the ex-Gaussian approach of estimating IIV based on research that suggests that the high IIV seen in children with ADHD is due to the increased amount of slow responses compared to controls (e.g., Buzy et al., 2009; Hervey et al., 2006; Leth-Steensen et al., 2000). Thus, the assumption is that τ captures the increased IIV due to lapses of attention, and as a result it would be the ideal metric when estimating IIV in a population that has a wide spectrum of attention impairment ranging from none to severe ADHD.

Based on the above literature review, the following hypotheses are proposed:

1. Ex-Gaussian parameter τ (IIV) will predict parent ratings of attention symptoms such that higher IIV will be related to a higher number of endorsed symptoms, but the parameters μ and σ, which represent the mean and standard deviation of the normal curve respectively, will not predict parent ratings of attention symptoms.

2. IIV will predict number of omission errors (suggesting inattention) but not commission errors (suggesting impulsivity) on an objective sustained attention task.

3. IIV will predict group membership (ADHD vs non-ADHD) above and beyond parent ratings of attention.

Methods

Participants

Participants were recruited from a combination of community settings and schools (School District 62: Sooke, and 63: Saanich) as a part of a larger study investigating impulsivity and motor activity in children with and without ADHD, which was approved by the University of Victoria Human Research Ethics Board. A total of 164 children were identified as potential study participants and 153 were able to be reached for determining eligibility.

Eligibility of child participants was determined using a screening interview (See Appendix A) that was completed over the phone with the child's parent/guardian. Criteria included children between 6 and 13 years of age who either had (1) a diagnosis of ADHD (2) difficulties with attention but no ADHD diagnoses, or (3) no difficulties with attention. Eligible children with ADHD who were on medication were asked to refrain from taking medication 48 hours before coming in for the study to avoid artifacts due to medication use (Kofler et al., 2013). The typical medication washout period in ADHD research often ranges between 12 to 48 hours (e.g, Bidwell et al., 2007; Biscaldi et al., 2016; Henríquez-Henríquez et al., 2015; Klein, Wendling, Huettner, Ruder, & Peper, 2006). All families were encouraged to speak with their child's doctor regarding medication concerns. Participants without a formal ADHD diagnosis were not on any medications.

Exclusionary criteria included children with complex medical history (e.g., cancer), neurological diagnoses (e.g., epilepsy, intellectual disability) and mental health diagnoses (e.g., Major Depressive Disorder, Generalized Anxiety Disorder). A co-morbid diagnosis of Learning Disability (LD) and Oppositional Defiant Disorder (ODD) were diagnostic exceptions for only the ADHD group due to the high co-morbidity between ADHD and these diagnoses (American Psychological Association, 2013; Tarver, Daley, & Sayal, 2014). Additionally, children with ADHD who were unable to refrain from taking medication (either due to longer acting medication, difficulty with initial titration, or discomfort with doing so) were ineligible for study participation. Following screening, a total of 104 participants (female = 36; age range = 6 – 13 years) went on to complete the study (See Table 1).

Assessment Measures

Parent/guardian measures.

Screening interview.

A screening interview, administered by trained research assistants to parents/guardians, was completed for each participant. This screener included eight questions regarding age, gender, grade, diagnoses (medical and mental health), and medication, to determine eligibility for the study (See Appendix A).

Demographic questionnaire.

Parents/guardians of eligible participants additionally completed a demographic questionnaire (See Appendix B) that included descriptive information such as ethnicity, language, and family income, as well as significant developmental history including medical, mental health and additional learning support services. This information was gathered to characterize the study sample.

Diagnostic interview.

A modified version of the Kiddie Schedule for Affective Disorders and Schizophrenia (K-SADS; J. Kaufman et al. (2016)) was completed with parents/guardians by research assistants trained in accurate use of the semi-structured interview and supervised by PhD level clinical psychology graduate students and/or lab supervisor Dr. Sarah Macoun. Parents were asked to rate the frequency of behaviours of their children while off medication (when relevant) on a three-point Likert scale ('Never', 'Sometimes', and 'Often'). The full ADHD module and ODD screener was completed by all participating parents/guardians; the full ODD module was only completed following a positive ODD screen. The K-SADS is a valid and reliable semi-structured interview aimed at determining diagnosis based on DSM-5 (American Psychological Association, 2013) criteria. This measure was used both as a confirmation of diagnostic status of participating children as well as determining level of attention difficulty in children without a formal diagnosis.

Attention and hyperactivity ratings.

Parents/guardians completed the ADHD Rating Scale-5 Home version (Child (5-10 years) or Adolescent (11-17 years); DuPaul, Power, Anastopoulos, & Reid (2016). This is a standardized rating scale based on DSM-5 ADHD diagnostic criteria that produces three symptom scores: Inattention, Hyperactivity/Impulsivity, and Total (Inattention plus Hyperactivity/Impulsivity). Parents/guardians were asked to rate their child's behaviours in the home environment over the past 6 months off medication. Ratings are on a four-point Likert scale ranging from 'Never' to 'Very Often'. A raw score is computed by summing the relevant items within each subscale. Internal consistency for the Inattention, Hyperactivity/Impulsivity, and Total scales for both age groups (child and adolescent) ranged from 0.89 to 0.96.

Executive function.

Parents/guardians completed the Comprehensive Executive Functioning Index (CEFI; Parent Scale; Naglieri & Goldstein (2013)) which is a norm-referenced measure of executive function abilities in children aged 5-18 years. Outcome scales on the CEFI include Attention, Inhibitory Control, Planning, Emotion Regulation, Initiation, Self-Monitoring, Flexibility, Organisation, and Working Memory. Internal consistency and test-retest reliability of the Parent Scale are 0.98 and 0.91, respectively.

Child participant measures.

In order to minimize the potential impact of learning difficulty and reading ability on participants' ability to understand and complete tasks, the measures administered did not require reading ability. Instructions were presented verbally, and examiners checked for understanding before beginning the task. Verbal responses were only required for the two subtests that comprise the Verbal composite of the intelligence test (See below).

Intellectual ability.

The Kaufman Brief Intelligence Test, Second Edition (KBIT-2; Kaufman & Kaufman, 2004) was used as an intellectual screening measure. It is a brief measure of general intelligence which consists of three subtests (two verbal, and one non-verbal) and produces age-based standardised composite scores in the verbal, and non-verbal domains which combine into a full-scale intelligence quotient (FSIQ).

Normative data (Standard Scores) on the KBIT-2 are available for ages 4-90 years. Internal consistency reliability scores for the 6-13 age group ranged from 0.86-0.93 for the Verbal composite, 0.81-0.89 for the Non-verbal composite, and 0.90-0.94 for the IQ composite. Test-retest reliability across the full normative age range (4-90 years) for the Verbal, Non-verbal, and IQ composite are 0.91, 0.93, and 0.90 respectively. The KBIT-2 IQ composite score is strongly correlated to the General Ability Index (0.84) and Full-Scale IQ (0.77) of the Wechsler Intelligence Scale for Children, 4th Edition (Homack & Reynolds, 2007).

Attention.

The Test of Attentional Performance for Children (KITAP; Zimmermann, Gondan, & Fimm, (2005)) sustained attention subtest (Ghost's Ball) was administered. The KITAP Ghost Ball is a 10-minute task where participants are required to monitor the appearance of ghosts on the screen. Participants are asked to respond by pressing a button only when ghosts of the same color appear consecutively. The task records number of omission errors, number of commission errors, and median RT in milliseconds. It consists of 300 trials (50 go-trials), with an interstimulus interval of 1500 milliseconds.

The Wack-a-mole is an experimental go/no-go computerized task which requires children to respond to target stimuli (by pressing a button) and to withhold that response when non-target stimuli appears (stimuli courtesy of Sarah Getz and the Sackler Institute for Developmental Psychobiology.) Baseline blocks are used to help participants develop a prepotent response to the stimuli, following which, test blocks are used to measure both the number of omission errors (i.e., no response for target stimuli) and commission errors (i.e. response to non-target stimuli). RT (in milliseconds) is recorded for all trials. RT trail-by-trial data was used for IIV data processing. Of note, the Wack-a-mole has 212 trials in total with 168 go trials and 44 no-go trials. The interstimulus interval is approximately 1160 milliseconds.

Procedures

Assessment.

Parents/guardians of participants were asked to provide informed consent to proceed with the study, and child participants were asked to assent to the same. Participants were informed that they are able to withdraw from the study at any time. Child participants completed a single one-on-one assessment with trained research assistants at the Child Development Lab, University of Victoria. A counterbalanced design was used to reduce order effects. The assessment lasted between two to two-and-a-half hours depending on the participant's need for additional breaks, which included a mandatory mid-testing 10-minute break. During the mid-testing break, participants were invited to choose a small $5 prize from a prize box, and at the end of the session they were rewarded with $10 in cash as well as an entry for a grand prize draw (iPad Mini).

While child participants were completing testing, their parents/guardians were interviewed using the K-SADS by trained research assistants, following which they independently completed the three questionnaires: Demographic questionnaire, ADHD Rating Scale-5, and CEFI. Parents/guardians were compensated with $10 cash for their time, and parking/transport fees were refunded where appropriate.

Data preparation.

Response times from the go/no-go measure (Wack-a-mole) were used to estimate IIV. Only response times from correct go trials were utilized (Note: incorrect go trials will have RTs of 0ms). Implausible outliers were then removed (i.e., extremely fast responses 200ms or less). Extremely slow responses (likely due to unintentional presses) were also removed. These limits were calculated separately for each participant such that the limit was established as three standard deviations above their mean. These filters resulted in an average of 163 trials per participant (range = 124 – 168).

The ex-Gaussian approach to estimating IIV was employed. Three ex-Gaussian parameters, mean (μ) and standard deviation (σ) of the normal component, and the combined mean and standard deviation of the exponential component (τ), was estimated for each participant using the open source program quantile maximum probability estimation (QMPE) software (Heathcote, Brown, & Cousineau, 2004). Response time distribution estimation was completed using quantile maximum probability (QMP) estimation, which combines maximum likelihood estimation and use of quantiles for RT grouping. That is, the RT data were grouped by quantiles before maximum likelihood estimation was completed; maximum likelihood estimation determines the parameters of a model, such that these estimated parameters maximize the likelihood that the data was actually observed (Heathcote, Brown, & Mewhort, 2002). QMP has been noted to be less biased and less variable than continuous maximum likelihood (CML) estimation, even when using RT sample sizes as small as 40 (Heathcote et al., 2002).

Results

Statistical Analyses

IIV parameters generated in QMPE (μ, σ, and τ) were imported into SPSS (v.23) where all analyses were completed. An alpha significance level of .05 (two-tailed) was used for all statistical tests. Before analysis, the data were examined for errors as well as univariate and multivariate outliers. No extreme (+3SD) outliers were present, with the exception of errors of commission on the sustained attention task, where seven outliers were removed from the control group. No multivariate outliers were present.

Group Assignment

Although participants were recruited as (1) children with ADHD, (2) children with attention problems but no ADHD, and (3) children with little to no attention problems, they were placed into two groups, 'ADHD' and 'Controls' (i.e., those who did not meet diagnostic criteria for ADHD) for some analyses (particularly the third hypothesis, See Objective and Hypotheses). Group assignment was based on the outcome of the K-SADS parent interview. This approach allowed participants to be placed in a group that best reflected their level of impairment (e.g., children reported as having severe attention problems, but for whom no formal diagnosis of ADHD was sought). Six children with a formal diagnosis of ADHD (N = 36), did not meet K-SADS criteria for an ADHD diagnosis and were therefore assigned to the Control group. Specifically, three children did not meet the minimum number of Inattention and/or Hyperactivity/Impulsivity symptoms, and three met the minimum symptom criteria but did not meet the criterion of having impairment in multiple settings such that parents indicated that the behaviours were only problematic in the home. Sixteen children without an ADHD diagnosis (N = 68) met K-SADS criteria for an ADHD diagnosis, and were thus assigned to the ADHD group. Within the KSADS-assigned ADHD group, 16 met criteria for the Inattentive presentation, six for the Hyperactive-Impulsive presentation, and 24 for the Combined presentation. Thus, final group assignment resulted in 58 children in the Control group, and 46 in the ADHD group.

Group Characteristics

For group comparisons, independent sample *t* tests were used for continuous variables (age, FSIQ, errors, RT metrics, and parent ratings). Pearson's χ^2 was used for categorical variables (gender, ethnicity, first language, other diagnoses, medication, and school support), however when underlying assumption were violated, Fisher's Exact test was used. The Mann-Whitney U test was used for the ordinal variable (family income).

Demographic comparisons and exact p-values for group comparisons are presented in Table 1. There were no significant age differences between the control (N = 58; mean age = 9.49 years, S.D. = 2.44 years, range = 6.00 – 13.90 years) and ADHD (N = 46, mean age = 9.56 years, S.D. = 2.21 years, range = 6.00 – 13.90 years) groups. There was also no group difference in ethnicity and first language. There was a significant association ($p < .05$) between group and gender with a smaller proportion of females in the ADHD group; there were 25 females in the control group (43.1%) and 11 in the ADHD group (23.9%). There was a significant difference ($p < .01$) between groups in family income such that the majority of the control group (59.1%) had a family income in excess of $100,000 while the majority of the ADHD group (71.4%) had a family income below $100,000. Regarding other diagnoses, there was no difference between groups on having a diagnosis of Oppositional Defiant Disorder (ODD), but there was significantly more participants ($p < .05$) in the ADHD group with a Learning Disability (LD) diagnosis (N = 4) compared to the control group (N = 0). There was a significant group difference on medication use ($p < .001$) such that 36.4% of children in the ADHD were currently on medication for attention difficulty whereas only 3.4% of children in the assigned control group were on medication. Regarding school supports, there was no significant difference between groups for gifted classes, speech language therapy, and occupational therapy. There was, however, significantly more participants in the ADHD group who received special education/LD classes ($p < .001$), behavioural adjustment ($p < .05$), tutoring ($p < .05$), counselling ($p < .05$), and social skills classes ($p < .05$).

Table 1. *Participant Demographic Information by Group.*

Demographic Variables	Control N=58	ADHD N=46	*P*
Age in years Mean (SD)	9.49 (2.44)	9.56 (2.21)	.883
Gender N Female (%)	25 (43.1)	11 (23.9)	.041*
Ethnicity N (%)[a]	European 31 (73.80) First Nation 0 (0.00) Asian 4 (9.50) African 1 (2.40) Mixed European/Asian 6 (14.30) Mixed European/African 0 (0.00)	European 31 (79.50) First Nation 1 (2.60) Asian 0 (0.00) African 0 (0.00) Mixed European/Asian 5 (12.80) Mixed European/African 2 (5.10)	**.103**
First Language N (%)[b]	English 43 (95.60) French 0 (0.00) Cantonese 2 (4.40) Portuguese 0 (0.00)	English 39 (95.10) French 1 (2.40) Cantonese 0 (0.00) Portuguese 1 (2.40)	**.266**
Family Income (%)[c]	0-40,000 (0.00) 40,001-75,000 (11.40) 75,001-90,000 (22.70) 90,001-100,000 (6.80) Over 100,000 (59.10)	0-40,000 (17.10) 40,001-75,000 (25.70) 75,001-90,000 (22.90) 90,001-100,000 (5.70) Over 100,000 (28.60)	.001**
Other Diagnoses N (%)[d]	Learning Disability 0 (0.00) ODD 0 (0.00)	Learning Disability 4 (8.50) ODD 1 (2.10)	**.032*** **.587**

Medication N (%)	None 56 (96.6) Biphentin[e] 1 (1.7) Intuniv[f] 0 (0.0) Concerta[e] 0 (0.0) Ritalin[e] 1 (1.7) Dexedrine[e] 0 (0.0) Strattera[f] 0 (0.0) Vyvanse[e] 0 (0.0) Combination[e] 0 (0.0)	None 28 (63.6) Biphentin[e] 6 (13.6) Intuniv[f] 1 (2.3) Concerta[e] 3 (6.8) Ritalin[e] 1 (2.3) Dexedrine[e] 1 (2.3) Strattera[f] 1 (2.3) Vyvanse[e] 1 (2.3) Combination[e] 4 (4.5)	.000***
School Support N (%)	Special Ed/LD Class 3 (5.30) Beh'l Adjustment 0 (0.00) Tutoring 4 (7.00) Gifted 2 (3.50) Counselling 15 (26.30) Speech Language 7 (12.30) Occupational 5 (8.80) Social Skills 4 (7.00)	Special Ed/LD Class 15 (31.90) Beh'l Adjustment 5 (10.60) Tutoring 10 (21.30) Gifted 2 (4.30) Counselling 22 (46.80) Speech Language 10 (21.30) Occupational 8 (17.00) Social Skills 12 (25.50)	.000*** .017* .036* **.588** .033* .228 .215 .010*

Note: SD = Standard deviation; * $p < .05$; ** $p < .01$; *** $p < .001$; **bolded text** = Fisher's Exact p-value; [a] 23 unanswered; [b] 18 unanswered; [c] 25 unanswered; [d] diagnosed by medical / psychology professional; [e] Stimulant; [f] Non-stimulant

Group comparisons (controls vs. ADHD) on performance measures and parent ratings are presented in Table 2. Groups significantly differed on general intelligence (K-BIT 2 FSIQ; t (102) = 2.04, *p* = .044), and errors of commission on the sustained attention task (t (45) = -4.12, *p* < .001, *d* = 0.89), however there was no significant difference between groups on errors of omission (t (97) = -0.46, *p* = .645) on the sustained attention task. Regarding overall performance on the go/no-go task (Wack-a-mole), there was no difference between groups on errors of omission (t (100) = -1.87, *p* = .065) or commission (t (76) = -1.67, *p* = .099).

Table 2. *Group Comparison on Performance Measures and Parent Ratings.*

Variables	Control (N = 58)	ADHD (N = 46)	*P*
K-BIT 2 FSIQ (StdS) Mean (SD)	109.12 (13.14)	103.59 (14.42)	.044*
μ Mean (SD)	395.48 (78.13)	390.74 (77.00)	.761

σ Mean (SD)	64.69 (28.18)	73.83 (33.84)	.140
τ Mean (SD)	161.27(71.08)	189.55 (70.53)	.049*
Sustained Attention Omission Errors Mean (SD)	9.12 (8.79)	9.93 (8.25)	.645
Sustained Attention Commission Errors Mean (SD)	5.10 (4.87)	18.67 (20.87)	.000**
Go/No-go Omission Errors Mean (SD)	2.48 (3.77)	4.52 (7.12)	.065
Go/No-go Commission Errors Mean (SD)	10.48 (6.17)	12.98 (8.33)	.099
Parent ADHD Rating Scale-5 (RS) Mean (SD)	5.91 (5.09)	18.76 (5.11)	.000**
Parent CEFI Attn (StdS) Mean (SD)	106.42 (15.06)	84.00 (11.33)	.000**
Parent CEFI Inhib (StdS) Mean (SD)	106.35 (15.05)	85.95 (13.19)	.000**

Note: * $p < .05$; ** $p < .001$; FSIQ = Full scale intelligence quotient; StdS = Standardized score; SD = Standard deviation; RS = Raw score; Attn = Attention; Inhib = Inhibitory Control;

Response time metrics were derived from performance on the Wack-a-mole task using ex-Gaussian analysis; there was no significant difference between groups on mean performance (μ; t (100) = 0.31, p = .761), or standard deviation (σ; t (100) = -1.49, p = .140). However, groups significantly differed on τ (t (100) = -2.00, p = .049, d = 0.40), an index of IIV commonly reported in the ADHD literature. Group differences in IIV were further demonstrated using a quantile-quantile plot (QQ-plot; See Figure 1). QQ plots are a graphical technique where τ of the ADHD group is plotted against τ of the control group to determine whether the two datasets come from a common distribution (i.e., proximity to 45-degree slope). Any deviation from the 45-degree slope indicates areas of the distribution where groups differ most, and if so, which group is more variable than the other. Recall that IIV estimates based upon τ represent the combined mean and standard deviation of the exponential component of the RT distribution (i.e., abnormally slow responses). Thus, Figure 1A suggests that children with ADHD differ from controls along virtually the entire τ distribution. Further, the fact that most values fall above the 45-degree slope indicates that children with ADHD have higher levels of IIV compared to controls for comparable points (quantiles) of the distribution.

Regarding parent ratings of inattention, groups significantly differed on both the CEFI ($t\ (97) = 8.45$, $p < .001$, $d = 1.68$) and ADHD Rating Scale-5 ($t\ (99) = -12.59$, $p < .001$, $d = 2.52$). There was also a significant group difference on parent ratings (CEFI) of Inhibitory Control ($t\ (97) = 7.07$, $p < .001$).

Figure 1. Quantile-Quantile Plot of τ Scores of the ADHD Group as a Function of τ Scores of the Control Group.

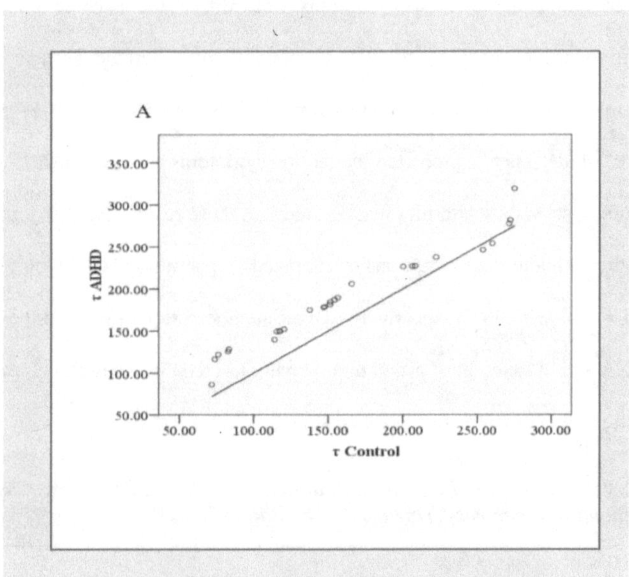

Hypothesis Testing

Predicting parent ratings of inattention symptoms.

Separate bivariate linear regressions were employed to determine the relationship between ex-Gaussian τ (IIV), μ, and σ, and the number of inattention symptoms endorsed on the parent version of the ADHD Rating Scale-5. Specifically, whole group analyses were conducted to determine whether τ, μ or σ (predictors) are independently able to predict the total raw score of inattention symptoms endorsed by parents (criterion). The ADHD Rating Scale-5 was used as the criterion variable because its items closely reflect the symptom criteria in the DSM-5, and it is completed independently by parents (i.e., not as a clinical interview).

Table 3 provides a summary of the regression values for variables predicting parent ratings of inattention symptoms. Regarding τ, the outcome of the regression analysis provided support that IIV significantly predicted the raw score of inattention symptoms as endorsed by parents (M = 11.63, SD = 8.18), $F(1, 97) = 5.30$, $p < .05$, with an R^2 of .05. That is, predicted inattention symptoms are equal to 7.05 + 0.03 (IIV). Figure 2 shows a scatterplot that summarizes these results. Neither μ nor σ significantly predicted inattention symptoms as endorsed by parents ($F(1, 97) = 0.52$, $p = .474$ & $F(1, 97) = 3.64$, $p = .060$, respectively). Bivariate interaction effects were explored between τ, μ, and σ as a function of group membership (ADHD vs Controls) on parent ratings of inattention. No interaction reached statistical significance.

Table 3. *Summary of Regression Analysis for Variables Predicting Parent Ratings of Inattention Symptoms Using the ADHD Rating Scale-5.*

Variable	B	SE B	β
IIV (τ)	.025	.011	.228*
μ	-.008	.011	-.073
σ	.049	.026	.190

Note: τ = Standard deviation of exponential component of response time distribution; μ = Mean of normal component of response time distribution; σ = Standard deviation of normal component of response time distribution; *$p < .05$

Figure 2. Scatterplot of IIV as a function of parent ratings of inattention on the ADHD Rating Scale-5

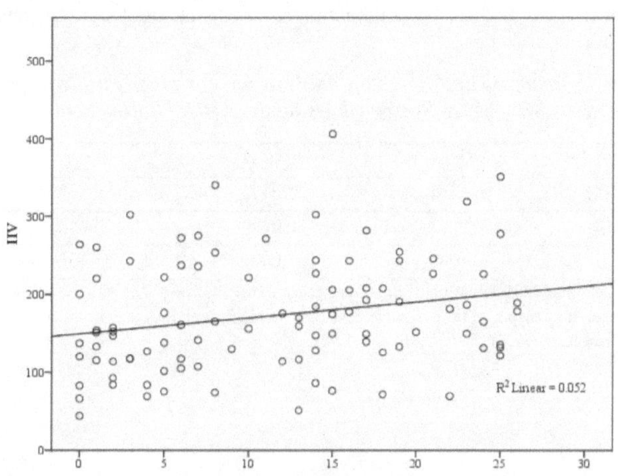

Additional analyses were done to determine whether ex-Gaussian parameters were predictive of parent ratings of hyperactive/impulsive symptoms given the relationship between inattention and hyperactivity/impulsivity. Of note, inattention and hyperactivity/impulsivity symptoms as rated by parents were significantly correlated $r(100) = .78, p < .001$. Table 4 provides a summary of the regression values for variables predicting parent ratings of hyperactive/impulsive symptoms. Regarding τ, the outcome of the regression analysis provided support that IIV significantly predicted the raw score of hyperactive/impulsive symptoms as endorsed by parents (M = 9.78, SD = 8.18), F (1, 97) = 14.93, $p < .001$, with an R^2 of .14. That is, predicted hyperactive/impulsive symptoms is equal to 2.55 + 0.04 (IIV). Figure 3 shows a scatterplot that summarizes these results. Additionally, σ significantly predicted hyperactive/impulsive symptoms as endorsed by parents (F (1, 97) = 11.69, $p < .01$, $R^2 = 0.11$) while μ did not (F (1, 97) =

1.60, $p = .210$). Bivariate interaction effects were explored between τ, μ, and σ as a function of group membership (ADHD vs Controls) on parent ratings of hyperactive/impulsive. No interaction reached statistical significance.

Table 4. *Summary of Regression Analysis for Variables Predicting Parent Ratings of Hyperactive/Impulsive Symptoms Using the ADHD Rating Scale-5.*

Variable	B	SE B	β
IIV (τ)	.041	.011	.367**
μ	.013	.011	.128
σ	.085	.025	.330*

Note: τ = Standard deviation of exponential component of response time distribution; μ = Mean of normal component of response time distribution; σ = Standard deviation of normal component of response time distribution; *$p < .01$; **$p < .001$

Figure 3. Scatterplot of IIV as a function of parent ratings of hyperactivity/impulsivity on the ADHD Rating Scale-5

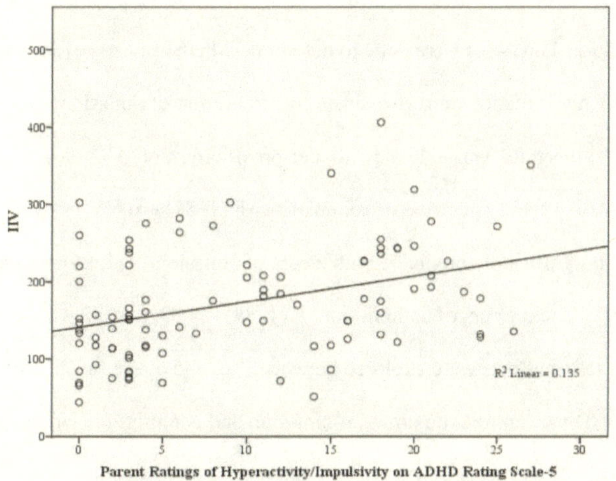

Predicting errors on a sustained attention task.

Separate bivariate linear regressions were employed to determine the relationship between τ (IIV) and errors of omission and commission on a sustained attention task (KITAP Ghost Ball). Specifically, whole group analyses were conducted to determine whether there was a relationship between IIV and errors using the entire spectrum of IIV (that is, low to high IIV regardless of group membership). Errors of omission (failing to respond to a stimulus) are considered to reflect lapses of attention, while errors of commission (responding when a response was not required) are likely due to inhibition failures. A summary of regression values is presented in Table 5.

The outcome of the regression analysis supports that IIV significantly predicted errors of omission (M = 9.53, SD = 8.55), F (1, 96) = 41.66, $p < .001$ with an R^2 of .30, but not errors of commission (M = 11.36, SD = 16.04), F (1, 88) = 3.78, $p = .058$. Additional analyses were done to determine whether mean (μ) and standard deviation (σ) of RT performance were also able to predict errors of omission and commission. Similar to IIV, mean RT was able to predict errors of omission, F (1, 96) = 22.10, $p < .001$ with an R^2 of .19, but not errors of commission, F (1, 88) = 0.67, $p = .416$. Standard deviation of RT significantly predicted both errors of omission, F (1, 96) = 43.87, $p < .001$ with an R^2 of .31, and errors of commission, F (1, 88) = 4.33, $p < .05$ with an R^2 of .05. Bivariate interaction effects were explored between τ, μ, and σ as a function of group membership (ADHD vs Controls) on errors of omission and commission. No interaction reached statistical significance.

Table 5. *Summary of Regression Analysis for Variables Predicting Errors of Omission and Commission on a Sustained Attention Task.*

Variables	Errors of Omission			Errors of Commission		
	B	SE B	β	B	SE B	β
IIV (τ)	4.46	0.69	.55**	0.05	0.03	0.20
μ	3.89	0.83	.43**	0.02	0.02	0.09
σ	1.83	0.28	.56**	0.14	0.07	0.22*

Note: * $p < .05$; ** $p < .001$

Predicting group membership based on full ADHD diagnostic criteria.

A binary logistic regression was employed to ascertain the effect of IIV on the likelihood that participants meet diagnostic criteria for ADHD. Group membership (ADHD vs Control) was assigned based on the KSADS parent interview such that participants were assigned to the ADHD group if they met full diagnostic criteria on the KSADS and the control group if they did not. There were no violations to the assumptions of the logistic regression. Results are presented in Table 6. The logistic regression was statistically significant, $\chi^2(1) = 3.949, p < .05$. For every unit increase in IIV, there is a 0.6% increased likelihood of being classified as ADHD. The model explained 5.1% (Nagelkerke R^2) of the variance in ADHD diagnosis and correctly classified 58.8% of cases with 79.3% specificity and 31.8% sensitivity.

Another logistic regression was employed to determine the effect of errors of omission on a sustained attention task (KITAP) on the likelihood that the participants meets diagnostic criteria for ADHD. Errors of omission were used as these are often interpreted in clinical practice as objective measures of lapses of attention. The logistic regression was not statistically significant, $\chi^2(1) = 0.217, p = .641$.

A third logistic regression was employed to determine the effect of parent ratings of attention on the likelihood that participants met diagnostic criteria for ADHD. The attention ratings of the CEFI were used because similar questionnaires are often completed by parents during an assessment of ADHD, the results of which can determine whether a full diagnostic interview may be warranted. There were no violations to the assumptions of the logistic regression. The logistic regression was statistically significant, $\chi^2(1) = 50.029, p < .001$. Overall, for every unit increase in CEFI Attention ratings, there is an 11.8% reduced likelihood of being classified as ADHD (recall that a higher score on the CEFI means better attention abilities as rated by parents). The model explained 53.1% (Nagelkerke R^2) of the variance in ADHD diagnosis and correctly classified 80.8% of cases with 81.8% specificity and 79.5% sensitivity.

A final logistic regression was employed to determine whether IIV improves the model when parent ratings of attention (CEFI) is included. The logistic regression was statistically significant, χ^2 (2) = 48.83, $p < .001$, however only parent ratings of attention contributed to the model. That is, IIV did not significantly improve the model. The model explained 52.6% (Nagelkerke R^2) of the variance in ADHD diagnosis and correctly classified 79.6% of cases with 81.8% specificity and 76.7% sensitivity.

Table 6. *Summary of Logistic Regression Variables*

Variable	B	SE B	Odds Ratio	Confidence Interval
Model 1:				
IIV	0.006*	0.003	1.006	1.000-1.011
Model 2:				
Errors of Omission	0.011	0.024	1.011	0.965-1.060
Model 3:				
CEFI Attn	-0.118**	0.023	0.889	0.849-0.930
Model 4:				
CEFI Attn	-0.118**	0.024	0.889	0.847-0.932
IIV	-0.001	0.004	0.999	0.991-1.007

Note: * $p < .05$; ** $p < .001$

Predicting group membership based on partial ADHD diagnostic criteria.

The above logistic regressions were repeated using partial diagnostic criteria for assigning group membership to ascertain IIVs ability to predict inattentive and hyperactive problems based on DSM-5s definition. Specifically, participants were re-assigned to groups (ADHD vs Controls) solely based on the DSM-5s ADHD diagnostic Criterion A. Individuals meet Criterion A if they have six or more symptoms of inattention and/or hyperactivity or impulsivity. Criteria B to E were disregarded as these criteria are not specific to attention difficulty but instead address aspects such as onset of symptoms and functional impact. This resulted in 51 participants being assigned to the ADHD group and 53 to the Control group based on the KSADS parent interview. Results were similar to when full diagnostic criteria were used and are reported in Table 6.

As with the full diagnostic criteria grouping, a binary logistic regression was employed to ascertain the effect of IIV on the likelihood that participants meet criterion A for ADHD, which specifically focuses on number of inattention and hyperactive/impulsive symptoms. There were no violations to the assumptions of the logistic regression. The logistic regression was statistically significant, $\chi^2 (1) = 6.936$, $p < .01$. For every unit increase in IIV, there is a 0.8% increased likelihood of being classified as meeting criterion A of an ADHD diagnosis. The model explained 8.8% (Nagelkerke R^2) of the variance in ADHD diagnosis and correctly classified 62.7% of cases with 73.6% specificity and 51% sensitivity.

The second logistic regression to determine the effect of errors of omission on a sustained attention task (KITAP) on the likelihood that the participants meets criterion A for ADHD was not statistically significant, $\chi^2 (1) = 1.151$, $p = .283$.

A third logistic regression was employed to determine the effect of parent ratings of attention (CEFI) on the likelihood that participants meet criterion A for ADHD. There were no violations to the assumptions of the logistic regression. As before, the logistic regression was statistically significant, $\chi^2 (1) = 60.914$, $p < .001$. Overall, for every unit increase in CEFI Attention ratings, there is a 13.9% reduced likelihood of being classified as ADHD (recall that a higher score on the CEFI means better attention abilities as rated by parents). The model explained 61.3% (Nagelkerke R^2) of the variance in ADHD diagnosis and correctly classified 81.8% of cases with 84% specificity and 79.6% sensitivity.

Finally, a logistic regression was employed to determine whether IIV improves the model when parent ratings of attention (CEFI) is included when predicting whether participants meet criterion A for ADHD. The logistic regression was statistically significant, $\chi^2(2) = 59.910, p < .001$, however only parent ratings of attention contributed to the model. That is, IIV did not significantly improve the model. The model explained 61% (Nagelkerke R^2) of the variance in criterion A and correctly classified 83.7% of cases with 84% specificity and 83.3% sensitivity.

Table 7. *Summary of Regression Variables Using Partial Diagnostic Criteria*

Variable	B	SE B	Odds Ratio	Confidence Interval
Model 1:				
IIV	0.008*	0.003	1.008	1.002-1.014
Model 2:				
Errors of Omission	0.026	0.024	1.026	0.976-1.076
Model 3:				
CEFI Attn	-0.139**	0.027	0.870	0.826-0.917
Model 4:				
CEFI Attn	-0.135**	0.027	0.873	0.829-0.921
IIV	0.002	0.004	1.002	0.993-1.011

Note: * $p < .05$; ** $p < .001$

Discussion

The current study examined the relationship between impairments in attention and IIV, as measured by the ex-Gaussian parameter τ, in a sample of children with a wide range of attention abilities ranging from typically developing to a formal ADHD diagnosis. The diagnostic utility of IIV in identifying children with ADHD was also assessed. Specifically, research has shown a relationship between IIV and attention abilities such that IIV is significantly higher in children with ADHD (See Kofler et al., 2013; Tamm et al., 2012). While there are multiple ways of estimating IIV, including ISD, ICV, and rISD, these methods have been criticized for various reasons including high influence of mean RT and an unclear theoretical interpretation (Hultsch et al., 2008). The current study used the ex-Gaussian approach to estimating IIV because of its clear link to the response distribution theory (Leth-Steensen et al., 2000) from which the current study follows, its removal of the influence of mean RT (Brown & Heathcote, 2003), and its recent increase in use in the ADHD literature (Adamo, Hodsoll, Asherson, Buitelaar, & Kuntsi, 2019; Epstein, Langberg, et al., 2011; Hervey et al., 2006; Kofler et al., 2013), including being proposed as a possible endophenotype of the disorder (Henríquez-Henríquez et al., 2015; Lin et al., 2015).

Although there has been increased research of IIV in children with ADHD, there is limited literature that directly examines the relationship between IIV and attention abilities across the attention spectrum using ex-Gaussian parameters; that is, is there a linear relationship between IIV, as measured by τ, and inattention symptoms in children? Thus, this study aimed to determine whether IIV was predictive of level of attention impairment across the entire spectrum of inattentive symptoms (none to severe ADHD) and, if so, whether it can also predict ADHD diagnostic status. Child participants completed a sustained attention task, which provided errors of omission and commission to represent inattentive and impulsive behaviors respectively, and a go/no-go task which provided response times that were used to estimate IIV. Parents completed a semi-structured interview to determine symptoms of inattention, hyperactivity/impulsivity, and ADHD diagnosis, as well as two non-diagnostic questionnaires to determine subjective ratings of inattention and hyperactive/impulsive symptoms in daily life.

Group differences (ADHD vs controls) in ex-Gaussian parameters were investigated prior to hypothesis testing. Recall that the ex-Gaussian approach assumes that there are two components of a response time distribution; (1) a normally distributed component (Gaussian) which is described by μ (mean of the normal distribution) and σ (standard deviation of the normal component) and (2) an independent exponential component (ex-) which represents the positive skew of the distribution due to a subset of abnormally slow responses and is described by τ (the combined mean and standard deviation of the skew). This positive skew (τ), or exponential component to the response time distribution, has been found to be greater in children with ADHD compared to controls based on a higher number of slow responses presumably caused by lapses of attention in the ADHD group (Adamo et al., 2019; Kofler et al., 2013; Leth-Steensen et al., 2000). On the other hand, central tendency estimates of the normal component of the distribution have been shown to be similar between groups, though this finding is inconsistent (See Kofler et al., 2013).

Current results using the ex-Gaussian approach show that children with ADHD have higher levels of IIV compared to controls such that groups differed on the exponential component of the response time distribution. These results support previous research using ex-Gaussian parameters that children with ADHD are more variable in their responses compared to controls based on a greater positive skew in their response time distribution (τ), but they are not necessarily slower overall (Epstein, Brinkman, et al., 2011; Kofler et al., 2013; Leth-Steensen et al., 2000; Vaurio et al., 2009). Thus, based on the theoretical relationship between τ and attention ability, this finding suggests that children with ADHD have a higher number of abnormally slow response times which is in keeping with the response distribution theory (Leth-Steensen et al., 2000). On the other hand, a more commonly used objective measure of inattention in clinical practice is errors of omission (Hall et al., 2016). Interestingly, current results found that groups did not differ on errors of omission on a sustained attention measure or on the go/no-go task on which IIV was estimated. Previous research on errors of omissions' ability to distinguish ADHD from controls are inconsistent, with some suggesting group differences exist (Berger, Slobodin, & Cassuto, 2017; Epstein et al., 2010; R. W. Y. Lee et al., 2015; Tarantino, Cutini, Mogentale, & Bisiacchi, 2013), and others suggesting no group differences (Christensen & Lundwall, 2018; Shaw, Grayson, & Lewis, 2005). In their study, Shaw et al. (2005) suggested that children with ADHD become more engaged on game-like tasks and show a reduced number of errors on these tasks compared to those that are not game-like in appearance. This may provide some explanation for the current study's lack of group difference on errors of omission since both the sustained attention and go/no-go tasks were game-like in their appearance (e.g., colorful, unique characters, story line, and background images). While it may be the case that game-like tasks are more engaging and likely reduce the amount of errors made by children with

ADHD, the current results uniquely highlight that children with ADHD have higher levels of IIV on a task where they perform no differently from controls. This suggests some clinical utility or sensitivity of IIV above errors of omission such that IIV is still able to discriminate between groups even when errors of omission cannot. This will be further discussed later within the context of predicting group membership.

While groups differed on IIV (τ), the current study found that groups did not differ on the normal components of the response time distribution (μ and σ) which suggests that children with ADHD are capable of responding just as quickly as children without ADHD. These results provide partial support for using the ex-Gaussian approach to estimate IIV, in keeping with the response distribution theory, compared to other methods such as ISD or ICV, which include the influence of both τ and σ in their estimates rather than separating their influence as the ex-Gaussian approach does. Thus, the ex-Gaussian approach allows for a more fine-tuned understanding of IIV. While some studies have reported similar results to those found here (Adamo et al., 2019; Galloway-Long & Huang-Pollock, 2018; Karalunas & Huang-Pollock, 2013) others have found group differences in μ and/or σ (Hervey et al., 2006; Hwang-Gu et al., 2019; Lin et al., 2015; Vaurio et al., 2009). These occasional findings are often attributed to differences in task parameters, particularly increased cognitive load or variations in interstimulus intervals, though no systematic investigation of this assumption has been undertaken (Hervey et al., 2006; Hwang-Gu et al., 2019; Lin et al., 2015; Tye et al., 2016; Vaurio et al., 2009). In general, elevations in μ have been thought to represent general slowing of RTs, while elevations in σ have been thought to represent deficits in motor timing and/or response preparation (Leth-Steensen et al., 2000; Vaurio et al., 2009). Given the task parameters used in the current study, the lack of group differences on μ and σ are likely due to engaging stimuli such that participants remained relatively engaged throughout the task or long interstimulus intervals which elicited lapses of attention and reduced demand on motor timing (Henríquez-Henríquez et al., 2015; Hervey et al., 2006; Leth-Steensen et al., 2000; Vaurio et al., 2009). It is also important to consider the composition of the groups here. Although participants were separated into two groups, ADHD and Control, recall that many children in the Control group had 'subthreshold ADHD' symptoms where they either did not meet the symptom cut-off or did not show impairment in multiple settings. This high number of attention problems in the control group can likely account for both the small effect size seen for τ, as well as lack of difference in σ. That said, while previous studies have found group differences in both the normal and exponential component of the RT distribution, τ has been found to consistently and reliably differentiate between groups (Hervey et al., 2006; Hwang-Gu et al., 2019; Lin et al., 2015). Overall, the current results as well as the consistency of IIV results in previous research (e.g., Hervey et al., 2006; Hwang-Gu et al., 2019; Kofler et al., 2013; Leth-Steensen et al., 2000; Lin et al., 2015; Vaurio et al., 2009), compared to components of the normal distribution, support the unique ability of IIV (τ) to distinguish between ADHD and controls, and provides some support for its utility in clinical settings.

The first hypothesis investigated the relationship between ex-Gaussian parameters and parent ratings of inattention. Specifically, does IIV, as represented by the ex-Gaussian parameter τ, significantly predict parent ratings of inattention symptoms based on a questionnaire designed to screen for ADHD symptoms, or simply, do inattentive behaviours increase with increases in IIV? The existence of such a relationship would provide support for additional analyses aimed at investigating IIVs utility in the diagnosis of ADHD. Relatedly, the first hypothesis also held that there would be no relationship between the mean and standard deviation of the normal component of the response time distribution, as represented by the ex-Gaussian parameters μ and σ, and parent ratings of inattention. The lack of such associations would further support the unique relationship between IIV and subjective reports of inattention and thus, the benefit of estimating IIV in clinical settings. Overall, the current study provided support for the first hypothesis such that IIV was significantly able to predict parent ratings of inattention, but μ and σ were not. These outcomes provide supporting evidence that IIV as measured by τ may be representative of lapses of attention, compared to μ or σ, such that as IIV can uniquely capture clinically meaningful lapses of attention that mean and SD cannot (Hervey et al., 2006; Leth-Steensen et al., 2000). An additional analysis was done to determine whether there was a main effect for group, that is, were the results mostly influenced by one group (ADHD or Controls). Results revealed that both groups (ADHD and Controls) equally contributed to these findings which suggests that the relationship between IIV and inattention is similar for both typically developing children and those with ADHD. The current results are similar to other studies investigating the relationship between IIV and parent ratings using different estimates of IIV including rISD in a mixed clinical sample (Ali, Macoun, Bedir, et al., 2019), and ICV in an ADHD sample (Gomez-Guerrero et al., 2011), as well as a recent investigation of τ in a pre-school sample (Hwang-Gu et al., 2019). One strength of the current results lies with the use of the ex-Gaussian parameters and the clear interpretation of τ capturing lapses of attention (Heathcote et al., 2002; Leth-Steensen et al., 2000). This finding is also particularly relevant for this age group because children are often identified for an ADHD diagnostic assessment during these school-years (American Psychiatric Association, 2013), and thus there is need for a reliable objective marker in this age group that is well supported in empirical research.

Given the relationship between inattention and hyperactive/impulsive symptoms and the importance of both these symptom dimensions in the diagnosis and clinical presentation of ADHD (American Psychiatric Association, 2013), additional analyses were conducted to investigate the relationship between ex-Gaussian parameters and hyperactive/impulsive symptoms as rated by parents. Results indicate that both IIV (τ) and σ are related to parent ratings of hyperactive/impulsive symptoms. Firstly, the association noted between σ and hyperactive/impulsive symptoms is in contrast to other studies that did not find such an association (Adamo et al., 2019; Hwang-Gu et al., 2019). Although ADHD and control groups did not differ on σ in the current study, it is not entirely surprising that σ, which is thought to represent motor timing and response preparation (Leth-Steensen et al., 2000; Vaurio et al., 2009), would be associated with hyperactive/impulsive behaviours as reported by parents. Secondly, an association between IIV and hyperactive/impulsive symptoms has been variably reported in the literature including IIVs association with both hyperactivity/impulsivity and inattention, using various metrics of IIV (Adamo et al., 2019; Gomez-Guerrero et al., 2011; Hwang-Gu et al., 2019; Kofler et al., 2013). Interestingly in a study with children with ADHD and co-morbid ASD, Adamo et al. (2019) found that IIV, as measured by τ, showed an association with hyperactive/impulsive symptoms but this association disappeared when the authors controlled for autism traits (e.g., social impairments, communication impairments, and restrictive and repetitive behaviours) suggesting that IIVs strongest association remained with inattentive symptoms. The current study's association between IIV and parent ratings of hyperactive/impulsive symptoms does not support the response distribution model of IIV in ADHD (Leth-Steensen et al., 2000) but, independently, it instead appears to be more in-line with the behavioural inhibition model (Barkley, 1997) which views behavioural inhibition as the core deficit in ADHD. However, since IIV as measured here was related to parent ratings of both inattention and hyperactivity/impulsivity it collectively implies a lack of specificity that may be due to the correlation between inattention and hyperactive/impulsive symptoms (Kofler et al., 2013). Thus, the next logical question is whether IIV is related to objective measures of inattention and/or hyperactivity/impulsivity in this population.

The second hypothesis sought to explore the relationship between IIV and objective performance on a sustained attention (CPT-type) task that is often used as a marker of attention deficits in clinical assessment settings (i.e., omission and commission errors). Specifically, the current study hypothesized that IIV would be significantly predictive of omission errors, but not commission errors. This would provide further supporting evidence of IIV as measured by τ, being related to inattention compared to impulsive behaviours on objective assessment measures. The results supported this hypothesis such that IIV was significantly able to predict omission errors but not commission errors. However, additional analyses revealed that IIV (τ) was not the only ex-Gaussian parameter uniquely related to omission errors. In fact, both μ and σ were significantly able to predict omission errors, while σ was the only parameter that was significantly able to predict commission errors. The current study's association between all ex-Gaussian parameters and omission errors had similar effect sizes (0.19-0.31) suggesting that lapses of attention (τ), general slowing of RTs (μ), and deficits in motor timing (σ) are similarly related to omission errors, while deficits in motor timing (σ) additionally contribute to commission errors.

The relationship between IIV and omission errors found in the current study is in-line with previous research which has proposed that both errors of omission and IIV share a common underlying mechanism; lapses of attention (Gmehlin et al., 2014; Tarantino et al., 2013). That is, brief lapses of attention likely lead to abnormally longer RTs (which contribute to τ), while longer lapses of attention result in a failure to respond to a target (which result in omission errors; Gmehlin et al., 2014). Relatedly, the relationship between μ and omission errors, and between σ and both error types is not unusual; however, the current results showing a positive relationship between μ and omission errors are in contrast to other studies (Lee et al., 2015; Tarantino et al., 2013). Lee et al. (2015) found a negative relationship between μ and omission errors, which they suggest represents a trade-off between speed and accuracy although this explanation better aligns with a negative relationship between μ and commission errors. Specifically, an increase in the speed of responding (lower RTs) would more likely result in impulsive responses (higher number of commission errors) rather than a failure to respond (higher number of omission errors). Having said that, the current study did not find a relationship between μ and commission errors, but rather a positive relationship between σ and commission errors.

Regarding the relationship found in the current study between σ and both errors of omission and commission, recall that σ is thought to represent deficits in motor timing or poor response preparation, which provides some explanation for its association with sustained attention errors such that poor timing can result in both omissions and commissions (Leth-Steensen et al., 2000; Vaurio et al., 2009). Indeed, Goetz et al. (2017) noted a relationship between motor symptoms, variability, and omission errors. On the other hand, the relationship between ex-Gaussian parameters and errors have been discussed to likely represent error monitoring, that is, pre- and post-error slowing which may have contributed to slower RTs, as well as variability in the normal and exponential components of RT (Epstein et al., 2010; Tarantino et al., 2013).

In sum, the outcomes of hypotheses one and two inconsistently align with the response distribution theory of IIV (Hervey et al., 2006; Leth-Steensen et al., 2000). Specifically, IIVs ability to predict both inattention and hyperactivity/impulsivity symptoms as rated by parents suggests that IIV may be related to both lapses of attention as well as poor behavioural inhibition. This interpretation is similar to the meta-analysis of IIV (using various metrics) that showed that while IIV is robustly associated with ADHD, it appears to lack specificity to underlying mechanisms and processes (Kofler et al., 2013) likely due to the strong association between inattention and hyperactive/impulsive behaviours. Thus, current results partially align with both the response distribution model based on IIVs association with parent ratings of inattention and omission errors (Hervey et al., 2006; Leth-Steensen et al., 2000) and the behavioural inhibition model based on IIVs association with parent ratings of hyperactivity/impulsivity (Barkley, 1997), although the results as a whole suggest a somewhat stronger association with the response distribution model. The discrepancy between objective performance (i.e., errors) and parent ratings is not uncommon in the ADHD literature where a disconnect is often noted for commission errors in particular;

that is, IIV as measured in the current study was related to parent ratings of hyperactive/impulsive behaviours but not commission errors (Sims & Lonigan, 2012). This suggests that commission errors may be less related to hyperactivity/impulsivity as seen in everyday life (Sims & Lonigan, 2012), and may be more closely related to motor timing/preparation as has been found in the current study. Finally, the finding that IIV was not the only parameter that predicted omission errors does not invalidate its association with lapses of attention, but instead suggests that omission errors may occur because of a combination of lapses of attention, RT slowing, and poor motor timing/regulation, while errors of commission are more likely related to poor motor timing/regulation.

One potential explanation for the mixed findings with respect to inattention and hyperactivity/impulsivity may be that the current study included participants with ADHD predominantly hyperactive/impulsive, predominantly inattentive, and combined presentations. Kofler et al. (2013) tentatively noted that the predominantly hyperactive/impulsive presentation of ADHD showed slightly higher levels of IIV (using various estimates of IIV), which could partially account for the association between IIV and parent hyperactive/inattentive ratings found in the current study. However, the current study also found greater associations between IIV and omission errors compared to commission errors, suggesting a greater association with objective performance of inattention compared to hyperactive/impulsive behaviours. Additionally, the finding that groups differed on IIV but not omission errors suggests that although IIV and omissions are related, IIV may be more sensitive to inefficiencies in attention and thus more clinically useful. While the current study did not directly assess the neural underpinnings of IIV, it is possible that there may be similar underlying neural mechanisms between IIV and inattention given the relationship between IIV and errors of omission found in the current study. Indeed, neuroimaging research has found an overlap between neural activity related to increased IIV as measured by τ and regions and/or networks associated with attention allocation including reduced deactivation of the DMN (Fassbender et al., 2009; Weissman et al., 2006), and reduced white matter integrity of fibers connecting attention related regions including the cingulum bundles (Lin et al., 2014) and superior longitudinal fasciculus (Wolfers et al., 2015). Regardless of the precise underpinning of IIV in ADHD, it remains that IIV has a robust association with the disorder and the results as discussed thus far provided support for investigating IIVs ability to predict diagnostic status within this sample.

The final hypothesis aimed to investigate IIVs ability to predict diagnostic status in a group of children with and without ADHD. Specifically, that IIV would predict diagnostic status above and beyond that of parent ratings. This analysis was especially important given the lack and inconsistent reliability of objective measures when diagnosing ADHD (Hall et al., 2016). As a result, ADHD is often diagnosed based on a combination of informant ratings and clinical interviews which are behaviorally defined and highly subjective (American Academy of Pediatrics, 2011). Thus, if IIV is able to improve the predictability of parent ratings when determining group membership then this would provide substantial support for its diagnostic utility.

Preliminary analyses were conducted before investigating this final hypothesis to determine whether IIV and errors of omission could independently predict group membership. The results found that IIV was indeed significantly able to predict group membership (ADHD vs Controls) while errors of omission did not significantly predict group membership. The inability of omission errors to predict group membership was not entirely surprising given the lack of group difference on omission errors. IIVs ability to predict group membership is similar to findings noted by Leth-Steensen et al. (2000) using receiver operating characteristic (ROC) methodology and ex-Gaussian parameters. However, while IIV was able to predict group membership in the current study, the accuracy with which it was able to do so was quite low such that only slightly more than half of participants (58.8%) were correctly identified in the model, with 31.8% sensitivity (true positives) and 79.3% specificity (true negatives). Specifically, in this case IIV appeared to be better at identifying participants without a diagnosis of ADHD compared to correctly identifying those with a diagnosis. Nevertheless, it was better than an objective measure often used in clinical practice; errors of omission on a CPT task.

IIVs limited sensitivity when predicting group membership may be associated with the inclusion of children with subthreshold impairment within the sample; that is, children with inattention and hyperactive/impulsive symptoms that fall short of meeting diagnostic criteria. Indeed, when follow-up analyses were done to predict group membership based on participants meeting criterion A of DSM-5s ADHD diagnostic criteria, that is, focusing solely on inattentive and hyperactive symptoms and ignoring whether participants met criteria B, C, D, and E (See Appendix C for diagnostic criteria), predictability slightly improved to 62.7%, while specificity decreased slightly to 73.6% and sensitivity increased to 51%. This improvement in sensitivity is likely reflective of IIVs ability to predict symptom criterion (i.e., severity of symptoms) but not additional, but required, diagnostic criteria such as age of onset and number of settings in which the symptoms prove problematic. Additionally, the gains on predictability when using criterion A only compared to full criteria provides some support for IIV capturing those children who fall into the 'zone of ambiguity' such that their symptoms are similar to those with an ADHD diagnosis, but they fail to meet full criteria (Parens & Johnston, 2009). Overall, these results firstly provide additional support to IIVs use in clinical settings as a marker of attention symptoms as outlined in DSM-5 criterion A, and secondly support the investigation of IIVs utility above and beyond parent ratings.

Results of the final hypothesis testing revealed that IIV failed to improve group predictability (using full diagnostic criteria) above and beyond parent ratings based on a questionnaire often used in clinical assessment settings. Specifically, parent ratings correctly identified 80.8% of cases, approximately 28% more than IIV alone. Both specificity and sensitivity were relatively high at 81.8% and 79.5%, respectively. Similar results were found when using partial diagnostic criteria (criterion A). The superiority of parent ratings can be explained firstly by considering the way ADHD is defined in the DSM-5 (See Appendix C). Specifically, ADHD diagnostic criteria are based on the subjective determination that the symptoms result in functional or developmental impairments with no objective guideline on how this should be determined thus producing a reliance on informants' opinion (American Psychiatric Association, 2013). Additionally, specific inattention and hyperactive/impulsive criteria are based on observable behaviours that cannot be captured by objective neuropsychological assessments (e.g., "Often does not seem to listen when spoken to directly"). Instead parent questionnaires are designed to capture these symptoms using multiple items that tap into situations where the behaviour may occur (e.g., CEFI items). Secondly, objective attention assessments have their own limitations when it comes to discriminating between children with and without ADHD. That is, they are often not ecologically valid in that they are completed in an artificial environment that does not emulate the environment observed by parents and teachers, and is thus not reflective of the symptom criteria needed for a formal ADHD diagnosis (Hall et al., 2016; Sims & Lonigan, 2012). Unfortunately, the results here add to the growing lamentations regarding a lack of objective measures that can improve upon the current methods of diagnosing ADHD (e.g., Hall et al., 2016; Sims & Lonigan, 2012; Tallberg, Råstam, Wenhov, Eliasson, & Gustafsson, 2019). However, there is still strong evidence for the utility of IIV in clinical settings, above that of omission errors, and particularly as a screener of general attention deficit in cases where there is a lack of access to informant ratings.

There are some limitations of the current study that need to be highlighted. Firstly, limitations associated with the sample used include gender differences, IQ differences, presentation type, and medication use. Specifically, the assigned ADHD and control groups were not matched on gender such that there were fewer females in the ADHD group compared to the control group. The higher proportion of males in the ADHD group is not entirely surprising given that the call for participants targeted children with a range of attention abilities (including difficulties with attention), and boys are more often identified as having attention problems by caregivers (American Psychiatric Association, 2013). However, research has highlighted that elevated IIV is independent of gender (Uebel et al., 2010), and controlling for gender in the current study did not impact the results reported here. Of note, although groups did not differ on age, controlling for age similarly did not affect the results.

The groups in the present study similarly differed on overall IQ such that the average IQ of the ADHD group was approximately 6 points lower than the control group. This difference in IQ between children with ADHD and typically developing children has been well documented in the literature, with some research suggesting a shared genetic relationship between IQ and ADHD (Frazier, Demaree, & Youngstrom, 2004; Kofler et al., 2013; Kuntsi et al., 2004). The group difference in IQ was highlighted in the current study to qualitatively describe the groups and the effect of IQ was not controlled for during hypothesis testing. The rationale for this comes from discussions surrounding the disadvantages of controlling for IQ in research of neurodevelopmental disorders (Dennis et al., 2009). This includes the assumption that IQ is confounded with and/or by the disorder thus the two groups (ADHD and Control) are not randomly assigned and controlling for IQ is inappropriate given the expected and pre-existing differences between these groups (Dennis et al., 2009). Dennis and colleagues (2009) also highlight the disadvantage of attempting to match groups based on IQ which results in either the ADHD group having a mean IQ that is higher than the population they represent or, conversely, the control group having a mean IQ that is below the mean of the population it represents.

The current ADHD sample also included all three presentations (predominantly inattentive, predominantly hyperactive/impulsive, and combined presentation) though the numbers within each group were small thus resulting in a lack of power that precluded an investigation of IIV within each presentation. A meta-analysis of IIV using multiple metrics tentatively proposed that IIV may be higher in individuals with a combined presentation (Kofler et al., 2013). The combined presentation was the largest presentation in the current study (N = 24) and this may have exerted some influence on the results. Future studies would benefit from a closer examination of IIV using the ex-Gaussian approach within each presentation of ADHD to determine whether IIV is more sensitive at detecting a particular presentation.

Finally, although data on medication use and type was collected for the larger study, the current study was not designed to test whether duration of medication use had any impact on IIV, as has been done in previous studies (e.g., pre and post-testing), or whether there is a difference in IIV between children with ADHD who have been medicated and those who are mediation naïve (Bédard et al., 2015; Epstein, Brinkman, et al., 2011; Ni et al., 2016; Spencer et al., 2009). In the current study, controlling for medication did not have an impact on the results though future studies may benefit from separating participants into groups based on medication type and duration to determine whether a significant relationship exists between treatment and IIV.

Secondly, there are some limitations to the ex-Gaussian method used in the current study. Specifically, while the ex-Gaussian method of estimating IIV has multiple strengths as discussed throughout the study, there are some limitations including the assumption that the RT distribution is skewed, which may not always be the case (Spencer et al., 2009). Additionally, the ex-Gaussian method has been criticized for its inability to determine the frequency at which these lapses of attention may occur, which may add valuable qualitative information when conceptualizing IIV (Helps, Broyd, Bitsakou, & Sonuga-Barke, 2011). Fast Fourier Transformations have been discussed as overcoming these limitations and a future direction for this area of research is a direct comparison of these methods in a population with a spectrum of attention impairments

(Helps et al., 2011; Karalunas, Huang-Pollock, & Nigg, 2013). Finally, if the ex-Gaussian method of estimating IIV were to be applied in clinical assessment settings it would require additional work on the part of the clinician. Currently, the clinician would be required to export the raw RT data, clean that data to remove incorrect responses and outliers, and then format the data for analysis by a separate software (e.g., QMPE). While this is complex and requires additional work, if IIV as represented by τ, were to be determined as a significantly useful addition to clinical work then CPT programs can be edited to include an algorithm that produces an estimation of τ. However, additional research is required before such an addition is justified.

Regarding effect sizes, a meta-analysis on IIV in ADHD reported moderate to large effect sizes though notably with much between study heterogeneity (Kofler et al., 2013). Relatedly, although there were variations in p-values in the current study, with some values marginally reaching significance, it is important to note that the effect sizes across analyses were similar with often overlapping confidence intervals. Effect sizes ranged from small to moderate, though it is important to note that even a small effect size can be meaningful where some researchers discuss the importance of interpreting effect sizes within the context of the research being conducted (Stukas & Cumming, 2014; Zakzanis, 2001). Additionally, classifying an effect size as small does not mean it is negligible as behaviour can be difficult to predict (Zakzanis, 2001) and a small effect size may have been observed due to various factors including the presence of attention problems in the control group and task type (e.g., larger effect sizes may be seen when using longer tasks with a greater number of trials to reliably detect IIV).

Regarding the tasks used in the current study, the sustained attention and go/no-go tasks are research-oriented and game-like tasks that are not typically used in clinical settings. While these tasks were specifically chosen to reduce the length of the overall test battery in the larger study and to improve participants' the level of engagement with tasks, they may have impacted the transferability of current findings into clinical settings. Additionally, as previously noted the type of tasks used can influence whether an effect is seen between groups as well as the size of the effect seen. As a result, future studies may benefit from an investigation of IIVs predictive ability when estimated from tasks regularly used in clinical assessment (e.g., Integrated Visual and Auditory (IVA) CPT) to determine if the current findings hold. Given the utility of these clinical tasks in assessing attention, IIV measured using these clinical tasks may be well-equipped to identifying children in the 'zones of ambiguity'.

Finally, while there is substantial research of IIV in ADHD (Kofler et al., 2013), the subject area may benefit from the development of normative data, including base rates, to facilitate the interpretation of IIV levels in clinical practice. It is important to highlight that use of this normative data may be limited to the specific method of IIV used to initially develop the normative data, though research with adults, and preliminary research with children, suggests that some metrics of IIV are comparable (Ali, Macoun, Halliday, et al., 2019; Stawski et al., 2019).

In sum, the current results suggest that IIV has a somewhat stronger association with inattention; that is, although IIV was non-specific in its association with parent ratings of ADHD symptoms (inattention versus hyperactive/impulsive), it did uniquely predict objective measures of inattention (omission errors) compared to hyperactive/impulsive behaviours (commission errors). This supports previous discussion that IIV is not specific to ADHD, as the relationship between IIV and attention was not solely driven by the ADHD group, and may instead be reflective of common symptoms of attention deficit that are also seen in other disorders such as ASD, FASD, depression and anxiety (e.g., Ali et al., 2017; Karalunas et al., 2014; Kofler et al., 2013). That said, IIV still proved to be useful in predicting group membership (ADHD versus Controls) in the absence of parent ratings, though parent ratings remained superior when available. Recent research has found that objective measures may be more useful when parent and teacher ratings are inconclusive and thus, IIV may be similarly useful in that regard (Tallberg et al., 2019). Notably, IIV as represented by τ in this sample appears to be more sensitive to DSM-5 Criterion A (Inattention and Hyperactive/Impulsive symptoms) compared to the full ADHD diagnostic criteria, which suggests that, compared to omission errors, IIV may be well suited to identifying children in need of additional ADHD diagnostic screening.

References

Adamo, N., Hodsoll, J., Asherson, P., Buitelaar, J. K., & Kuntsi, J. (2019). Ex-Gaussian, frequency and reward analyses reveal specificity of reaction time fluctuations to ADHD and not Autism traits. *Journal of Abnormal Child Psychology*, *47*(3), 557–567. https://doi.org/10.1007/s10802-018-0457-z

Adamo, N., Huo, L., Adelsberg, S., Petkova, E., Castellanos, F. X., & Di Martino, A. (2014). Response time intra-subject variability: Commonalities between children with autism spectrum disorders and children with ADHD. *European Child & Adolescent Psychiatry*, *23*(2), 69–79. https://doi.org/10.1007/s00787-013-0428-4

Adams, Z. W., Roberts, W. M., Milich, R., & Fillmore, M. T. (2011). Does response variability predict distractibility among adults with attention-deficit/hyperactivity disorder? *Psychological Assessment*, *23*(2), 427–436. https://doi.org/10.1037/a0022112

Adleman, N. E., Chen, G., Reynolds, R. C., Frackman, A., Razdan, V., Weissman, D. H., … Leibenluft, E. (2016). Age-related differences in the neural correlates of trial-to-trial variations of reaction time. *Developmental Cognitive Neuroscience*, *19*, 248–257. https://doi.org/10.1016/j.dcn.2016.05.001

Albaugh, M. D., Orr, C., Chaarani, B., Althoff, R. R., Allgaier, N., D'Alberto, N., … Potter, A. S. (2016). Inattention and reaction time variability are linked to ventromedial prefrontal volume in adolescents. *Biological Psychiatry*, *82*(9), 660–668. https://doi.org/10.1016/j.biopsych.2017.01.003

Ali, S., Kerns, K. A., Mulligan, B. P., Olson, H. C., & Astley, S. J. (2017). An investigation of intra-individual variability in children with fetal alcohol spectrum disorder (FASD). *Child Neuropsychology*, *24*(5), 617–637. https://doi.org/10.1080/09297049.2017.1302579

Ali, S., Macoun, S. J., Bedir, B., & MacDonald, S. W. S. (2019). Intraindividual variability in children is related to informant ratings of attention and executive function. *Journal of Clinical and Experimental Neuropsychology*, *41*(7), 740–748. https://doi.org/10.1080/13803395.2019.1617249

Ali, S., Macoun, S. J., Halliday, D. W. R., MacDonald, S. W. S., Kim, A. Y., & Krauss, M. W. R. (2019). Comparing operationalizations of intraindividual variability in a child population: Eenie, Meenie, Miney, but maybe not Mo [Abstract]. *Journal of the International Neuropsychological Society*, *25*(S1), 53–54.

American Academy of Pediatrics. (2011). ADHD: Clinical practice guideline for the diagnosis, evaluation, and treatment of Attention-Deficit/Hyperactivity Disorder in children and adolescents. *Pediatrics*, *128*(5), 1007–1022. https://doi.org/10.1542/peds.2011-2654

American Psychiatric Association. (2013). *Diagnostic and statistical manual of mental disorders* (5th ed.). Arlington, VA: American Psychiatric Association.

Antonini, T. N., Narad, M. E., Langberg, J. M., & Epstein, J. N. (2013). Behavioral correlates of reaction time variability in children with and without ADHD. *Neuropsychology*, *27*(2), 201–209. https://doi.org/10.1037/a0032071

Barkley, R. a. (1997). Behavioral inhibition, sustained attention, and executive functions: constructing a unifying theory of ADHD. *Psychological Bulletin*, *121*(1), 65–94. https://doi.org/10.1037/0033-2909.121.1.65

Beaulieu-Bonneau, S., Fortier-Brochu, É., Ivers, H., & Morin, C. M. (2017). Attention following traumatic brain injury: Neuropsychological and driving simulator data, and association with sleep, sleepiness, and fatigue. *Neuropsychological Rehabilitation*, *27*(2), 216–238. https://doi.org/10.1080/09602011.2015.1077145

Bédard, A. C. V, Stein, M. A., Halperin, J. M., Krone, B., Rajwan, E., & Newcorn, J. H. (2015). Differential impact of methylphenidate and atomoxetine on sustained attention in youth with attention-deficit/hyperactivity disorder. *Journal of Child Psychology and Psychiatry and Allied Disciplines*, *56*(1), 40–48. https://doi.org/10.1111/jcpp.12272

Bellgrove, M. A., Hester, R., & Garavan, H. (2004). The functional neuroanatomical correlates of response variability: Evidence from a response inhibition task. *Neuropsychologia*, *42*(14), 1910–1916. https://doi.org/10.1016/j.neuropsychologia.2004.05.007

Berger, I., Slobodin, O., & Cassuto, H. (2017). Usefulness and validity of continuous performance tests in the diagnosis of attention-deficit hyperactivity disorder children. *Archives of Clinical Neuropsychology*, *32*(1), 81–93. https://doi.org/10.1093/arclin/acw101

Bharath, S., Sadanand, S., Kumar, K. J., Balachandar, R., Joshi, H., & Varghese, M. (2017). Clinical and neuropsychological profile of persons with mild cognitive impairment, a hospital based study from a lower and middle income country. *Asian Journal of Psychiatry*, *30*(2017), 185–189. https://doi.org/10.1016/j.ajp.2017.10.007

Bidwell, L. C., Willcutt, E. G., DeFries, J. C., & Pennington, B. F. (2007). Testing for neuropsychological endophenotypes in siblings discordant for Attention-Deficit/Hyperactivity Disorder. *Biological Psychiatry*, *62*(9), 991–998. https://doi.org/10.1016/j.biopsych.2007.04.003

Bielak, A. A. M., Cherbuin, N., Bunce, D., & Anstey, K. J. (2014). Intraindividual variability is a fundamental phenomenon of aging: Evidence from an 8-year longitudinal study across young, middle, and older adulthood. *Developmental Psychology*, *50*(1), 143–151. https://doi.org/10.1037/a0032650

Bielak, A. a M., Hultsch, D. F., Strauss, E., MacDonald, S. W. S., & Hunter, M. a. (2010). Intraindividual variability in reaction time predicts cognitive outcomes 5 years later. *Neuropsychology*, *24*(6), 731–741. https://doi.org/10.1037/a0019802

Biscaldi, M., Bednorz, N., Weissbrodt, K., Saville, C. W. N., Feige, B., Bender, S., & Klein, C. (2016). Cognitive endophenotypes of attention deficit/hyperactivity disorder and intra-subject variability in patients with autism spectrum disorder. *Biological Psychology*, *118*, 25–34. https://doi.org/10.1016/j.biopsycho.2016.04.064

Borella, E., Chicherio, C., Re, A. M., Sensini, V., & Cornoldi, C. (2011). Increased intraindividual variability is a marker of ADHD but also of dyslexia: A study on handwriting. *Brain and Cognition*, *77*(1), 33–39. https://doi.org/10.1016/j.bandc.2011.06.005

Brennan, A. A., Bruderer, A. J., Liu-Ambrose, T., Handy, T. C., & Enns, J. T. (2017). Lifespan changes in attention revisited: Everyday visual search. *Canadian Journal of Experimental Psychology/Revue Canadienne de Psychologie Expérimentale*, *71*(2), 160–171. https://doi.org/10.1037/cep0000130

Brown, S., & Heathcote, A. (2003). QMLE: Fast, robust, and efficient estimation of distribution functions based on quantiles. *Behavior Research Methods, Instruments, & Computers : A Journal of the Psychonomic Society, Inc*, *35*(4), 485–492. https://doi.org/10.3758/BF03195527

Bunce, D., Anstey, K. J., Cherbuin, N., Burns, R., Christensen, H., Wen, W., & Sachdev, P. S. (2010). Cognitive deficits are associated with frontal and temporal lobe white matter lesions in middle-aged adults living in the community. *PLoS ONE*, *5*(10). https://doi.org/10.1371/journal.pone.0013567

Bunce, D., Anstey, K. J., Christensen, H., Dear, K., Wen, W., & Sachdev, P. (2007). White matter hyperintensities and within-person variability in community-dwelling adults aged 60-64 years. *Neuropsychologia*, *45*(9), 2009–2015. https://doi.org/10.1016/j.neuropsychologia.2007.02.006

Burd, L. (2016). FASD and ADHD: Are they related and how? *BMC Psychiatry*, *16*(1), 1–4. https://doi.org/10.1186/s12888-016-1028-x

Burton, C. L., Strauss, E., Hultsch, D. F., Moll, A., & Hunter, M. a. (2006). Intraindividual variability as a marker of neurological dysfunction: a comparison of Alzheimer's disease and Parkinson's disease. *Journal of Clinical and Experimental Neuropsychology*, *28*(1), 67–83. https://doi.org/10.1080/13803390490918318

Bush, G. (2011). Cingulate, frontal, and parietal cortical dysfunction in attention-deficit/hyperactivity disorder. *Biological Psychiatry*, *69*(12), 1160–1167. https://doi.org/10.1016/j.biopsych.2011.01.022

Buzy, W. M., Medoff, D. R., & Schweitzer, J. B. (2009). Intra-individual variability among children with ADHD on a working memory task: An ex-Gaussian approach. *Child Neuropsychology : A Journal on Normal and Abnormal Development in Childhood and Adolescence*, *15*(5), 441–459. https://doi.org/10.1080/09297040802646991

Castellanos, F. X., Kelly, C., & Milham, M. P. (2009). The restless brain: Attention-deficit hyperactivity disorder, resting-state functional connectivity, and intrasubject variability. *Canadian Journal of Psychiatry*, *54*(10), 665–672.

Castellanos, F. X., & Proal, E. (2012). Large-scale brain systems in ADHD: Beyond the prefrontal-striatal model. *Trends in Cognitive Sciences*, *16*(1), 17–26. https://doi.org/10.1016/j.tics.2011.11.007

Castellanos, F. X., Sonuga-Barke, E. J. S., Milham, M. P., & Tannock, R. (2006). Characterizing cognition in ADHD: Beyond executive dysfunction. *Trends in Cognitive Sciences*, *10*(3). https://doi.org/10.1016/j.tics.2006.01.011

Castellanos, F. X., & Tannock, R. (2002). Neuroscience of attention-deficit/hyperactivity disorder: The search for endophenotypes. *Nature Reviews. Neuroscience*, *3*(8), 617–628. https://doi.org/10.1038/nrn896

Chen, L., Hu, X., Ouyang, L., He, N., Liao, Y., Liu, Q., … Gong, Q. (2016). A systematic review and meta-analysis of tract-based spatial statistics studies regarding attention-deficit/hyperactivity disorder. *Neuroscience and Biobehavioral Reviews*, *68*(37), 838–847. https://doi.org/10.1016/j.neubiorev.2016.07.022

Cheung, C. H. M., McLoughlin, G., Brandeis, D., Banaschewski, T., Asherson, P., & Kuntsi, J. (2017). Neurophysiological correlates of attentional fluctuation in Attention-Deficit/Hyperactivity Disorder. *Brain Topography*, *30*(3), 1–13. https://doi.org/10.1007/s10548-017-0554-2

Cho, S.-C., Kim, J.-W., Kim, B.-N., Hwang, J.-W., Park, M., Kim, S. A., … Park, T.-W. (2008). Possible association of the alpha-2A-adrenergic receptor gene with response time variability in attention deficit hyperactivity disorder. *American Journal of Medical Genetics. Part B, Neuropsychiatric Genetics : The Official Publication of the International Society of Psychiatric Genetics*, *147B*(6), 957–963. https://doi.org/10.1002/ajmg.b.30725

Christensen, K. E., & Lundwall, R. A. (2018). Errors on a computer task and subclinical symptoms of attention-deficit/hyperactivity disorder (ADHD). *Scandinavian Journal of Psychology*, *59*(5), 511–517. https://doi.org/10.1111/sjop.12462

Coghill, D. R., Banaschewski, T., Soutullo, C., Cottingham, M. G., & Zuddas, A. (2017). Systematic review of quality of life and functional outcomes in randomized placebo-controlled studies of medications for attention-deficit/hyperactivity disorder. *European Child & Adolescent Psychiatry*, *26*(11), 1283–1307. https://doi.org/10.1007/s00787-017-0986-y

Cole, W. R., Gregory, E., Arrieux, J. P., & Haran, F. J. (2017). Intra-individual cognitive variability: An examination of ANAM4 TBI-MIL simple reaction time data from service members with and without mild traumatic brain injury. *Journal of the International Neuropsychological Society*, *24*(2), 156–162. https://doi.org/10.1017/S1355617717000856

Cubillo, A., Halari, R., Smith, A., Taylor, E., & Rubia, K. (2012). A review of fronto-striatal and fronto-cortical brain abnormalities in children and adults with Attention Deficit Hyperactivity Disorder (ADHD) and new evidence for dysfunction in adults with ADHD during motivation and attention. *Cortex*, *48*(2), 194–215. https://doi.org/10.1016/j.cortex.2011.04.007

Dennis, M., Francis, D. J., Cirino, P. T., Schachar, R., Barnes, M. A., & Fletcher, J. M. J. M. (2009). Why IQ is not a covariate in cognitive studies of neurodevelopmental disorders. *Journal of the International Neuropsychological Society*, *15*(3), 331–343.

https://doi.org/10.1017/S1355617709090481

Dinstein, I., Heeger, D. J., & Behrmann, M. (2015). Neural variability: Friend or foe? *Trends in Cognitive Sciences*, *19*(6), 322–328. https://doi.org/10.1016/j.tics.2015.04.005

Doernberg, E., & Hollander, E. (2016). Neurodevelopmental Disorders (ASD and ADHD): DSM-5, ICD-10, and ICD-11. *CNS Spectrums*, *21*(4), 295–299. https://doi.org/10.1017/S1092852916000262

DuPaul, G. J., Power, T. J., Anastopoulos, A. D., & Reid, R. (2016). *ADHD Rating Scale-5 for children and adolescents: Checklists, norms, and clinical interpretation.* New York, NY: The Guilford Press.

Durston, S., Van Belle, J., & De Zeeuw, P. (2011). Differentiating frontostriatal and fronto-cerebellar circuits in attention-deficit/hyperactivity disorder. *Biological Psychiatry*, *69*(12), 1178–1184. https://doi.org/10.1016/j.biopsych.2010.07.037

Dykiert, D., Der, G., Starr, J. M., & Deary, I. J. (2012). Age differences in intra-individual variability in simple and choice reaction time: Systematic review and meta-analysis. *PLoS ONE*, *7*(10), 1–23. https://doi.org/10.1371/journal.pone.0045759

Elia, J., Ambrosini, P., & Berrettini, W. (2008). ADHD characteristics: I. Concurrent co-morbidity patterns in children and adolescents. *Child and Adolescent Psychiatry and Mental Health*, *2*(15), 1–9. https://doi.org/10.1186/1753-2000-2-Received

Epstein, J. N., Brinkman, W. B., Froehlich, T., Langberg, J. M., Narad, M. E., Antonini, T. N., … Altaye, M. (2011). Effects of stimulant medication, incentives, and event rate on reaction time variability in children with ADHD. *Neuropsychopharmacology*, *36*(5), 1060–1072. https://doi.org/10.1038/npp.2010.243

Epstein, J. N., Hwang, M. E., Antonini, T. N., Langberg, J. M., Altaye, M., & Arnold, E. L. (2010). Examining predictors of reaction times in children with ADHD and normal controls. *Journal of the International Neuropsychological Society*, *16*(01), 138–147. https://doi.org/10.1017/S1355617709991111

Epstein, J. N., Langberg, J. M., Rosen, P. J., Graham, A., Narad, M. E., Antonini, T. N., … Altaye, M. (2011). Evidence for higher reaction time variability for children with ADHD on a range of cognitive tasks including reward and event rate manipulations. *Neuropsychology*, *25*(4), 427–441. https://doi.org/10.1037/a0022155

Evans, S. W., Owens, J. S., & Bunford, N. (2014). Evidence-based psychosocial treatments for children and adolescents with Attention-Deficit/Hyperactivity Disorder. *Journal of Clinical Child & Adolescent Psychology*, *43*(4), 527–551. https://doi.org/10.1080/15374416.2013.850700

Faraone, S. V., Perlis, R. H., Doyle, A. E., Smoller, J. W., Goralnick, J. J., Holmgren, M. A., & Sklar, P. (2005). Molecular genetics of attention-deficit/hyperactivity disorder. *Biological Psychiatry*, *57*(11), 1313–1323.

https://doi.org/10.1016/j.biopsych.2004.11.024

Fassbender, C., Zhang, H., Buzy, W. M., Cortes, C. R., Mizuiri, D., Beckett, L., & Schweitzer, J. B. (2009). A lack of default network suppression is linked to increased distractibility in ADHD. *Brain Research*, *1273*, 114–128. https://doi.org/10.1016/j.brainres.2009.02.070

Findling, R. L. (2008). Evolution of the treatment of attention-deficit/hyperactivity disorder in children: A review. *Clinical Therapeutics*, *30*(5), 942–957. https://doi.org/10.1016/j.clinthera.2008.05.006

Ford-Jones, P. C. (2015). Misdiagnosis of attention deficit hyperactivity disorder: "Normal behaviour" and relative maturity. *Pediatric Child Health*, *20*(4), 200–203.

Frazier-Wood, A. C., Bralten, J., Arias-Vasquez, A., Luman, M., Ooterlaan, J., Sergeant, J., … Rommelse, N. N. J. (2012). Neuropsychological intra-individual variability explains unique genetic variance of ADHD and shows suggestive linkage to chromosomes 12, 13, and 17. *American Journal of Medical Genetics, Part B: Neuropsychiatric Genetics*, *159 B*(2), 131–140. https://doi.org/10.1002/ajmg.b.32018

Frazier, T. W., Demaree, H. A., & Youngstrom, E. A. (2004). Meta-analysis of intellectual and neuropsychological test performance in attention-deficit/hyperactivity disorder. *Neuropsychology*, *18*(3), 543–555. https://doi.org/10.1037/0894-4105.18.3.543

Friedman, L. A., & Rapoport, J. L. (2015). Brain development in ADHD. *Current Opinion in Neurobiology*, *30*, 106–111. https://doi.org/10.1016/j.conb.2014.11.007

Froehlich, T., Lanphear, B. P., Auinger, P., Hornung, R., Epstein, J. N., Braun, J., & Kahn, R. S. (2009). Association of tobacco and lead exposures with Attention-Deficit/Hyperactivity Disorder. *Pediatrics*, *124*(6), e1054–e1063. https://doi.org/10.1542/peds.2009-0738.

Galloway-Long, H., & Huang-Pollock, C. (2018). Using inspection time and ex-Gaussian parameters of reaction time to predict executive functions in children with ADHD. *Intelligence*, *69*, 186–194. https://doi.org/10.1016/j.intell.2018.06.005

Gargaro, B. A., Rinehart, N. J., Bradshaw, J. L., Tonge, B. J., & Sheppard, D. M. (2011). Autism and ADHD: How far have we come in the comorbidity debate? *Neuroscience and Biobehavioral Reviews*, *35*(5), 1081–1088. https://doi.org/10.1016/j.neubiorev.2010.11.002

Garrett, D. D., Samanez-Larkin, G. R., MacDonald, S. W. S., Lindenberger, U., McIntosh, A. R., & Grady, C. L. (2013). Moment-to-moment brain signal variability: A next frontier in human brain mapping? *Neuroscience and Biobehavioral Reviews*, *37*(4), 610–624. https://doi.org/10.1016/j.neubiorev.2013.02.015

Gmehlin, D., Fuermaier, A. B. M., Walther, S., Debelak, R., Rentrop, M., Westermann, C., … Aschenbrenner, S. (2014). Intraindividual variability in inhibitory function in adults with ADHD – An ex-Gaussian approach. *PLoS ONE*, *9*(12), e112298. https://doi.org/10.1371/journal.pone.0112298

Goetz, M., Schwabova, J., Hlavka, Z., Ptacek, R., Zumrova, A., Hort, V., & Doyle, R. (2017). Cerebellar symptoms are associated with omission errors and variability of response time in children with ADHD. *Journal of Attention Disorders*, *21*(3), 190–199. https://doi.org/10.1177/1087054713517745

Gomez-Guerrero, L., Martin, C. D., Mairena, M. A., Di Martino, A., Wang, J., Mendelsohn, A. L., … Castellanos, F. X. (2011). Response-time variability is related to parent ratings of inattention, hyperactivity, and executive function. *Journal of Attention Disorders*, *15*(7), 572–582. https://doi.org/10.1177/1087054709356379

Gonen-Yaacovi, G., Arazi, A., Shahar, N., Karmon, A., Haar, S., Meiran, N., & Dinstein, I. (2016). Increased ongoing neural variability in ADHD. *Cortex*, *81*, 50–63. https://doi.org/10.1016/j.cortex.2016.04.010

Goodlad, J. K., Marcus, D. K., & Fulton, J. J. (2013). Lead and Attention-Deficit/Hyperactivity Disorder (ADHD) symptoms: A meta-analysis. *Clinical Psychology Review*, *33*(3), 417–425. https://doi.org/10.1016/j.cpr.2013.01.009

Greven, C. U., Bralten, J., Mennes, M., O'Dwyer, L., Van Hulzen, K. J. E., Rommelse, N., … Buitelaar, J. K. (2015). Developmentally stable whole-brain volume reductions and developmentally sensitive caudate and putamen volume alterations in those with attention-deficit/hyperactivity disorder and their unaffected siblings. *JAMA Psychiatry*, *72*(5), 490–499. https://doi.org/10.1001/jamapsychiatry.2014.3162

Grizenko, N., Fortier, M.-E., Gaudreau-Simard, M., Jolicoeur, C., & Joober, R. (2015). The effect of maternal stress during pregnancy on IQ and ADHD symptomatology. *Journal of the Canadian Academy of Child and Adolescent Psychiatry*, *24*(2), 92–99.

Grizenko, N., Fortier, M. E., Zadorozny, C., Thakur, G., Schmitz, N., Duval, R., & Joober, R. (2012). Maternal stress during pregnancy, ADHD symptomatology in children and genotype: Gene-environment interaction. *Journal of the Canadian Academy of Child and Adolescent Psychiatry*, *21*(1), 9–15.

Haack, L. M., Villodas, M. T., Mcburnett, K., Hinshaw, S., & Pfiffner, L. J. (2016). Parenting mediates symptoms and impairment in children with ADHD-inattentive type. *Journal of Clinical Child & Adolescent Psychology*, *45*(2), 155–166. https://doi.org/10.1080/15374416.2014.958840

Hall, C. L., Valentine, A. Z., Groom, M. J., Walker, G. M., Sayal, K., Daley, D., & Hollis, C. (2016). The clinical utility of the continuous performance test and objective measures of activity for diagnosing and monitoring ADHD in children: A systematic review. *European Child and Adolescent Psychiatry*, *25*(7), 677–699. https://doi.org/10.1007/s00787-015-0798-x

Halperin, J. M., Bédard, A. C. V, & Curchack-Lichtin, J. T. (2012). Preventive interventions for ADHD: A neurodevelopmental perspective. *Neurotherapeutics*, *9*(3), 531–541. https://doi.org/10.1007/s13311-012-0123-z

Hanwella, R., Senanayake, M., & de Silva, V. (2011). Comparative efficacy and acceptability of methylphenidate and atomoxetine in treatment of attention deficit hyperactivity disorder in children and adolescents: a meta-analysis. *BMC Psychiatry*, *11*(1), 176. https://doi.org/10.1186/1471-244X-11-176

Haynes, B. I., Bauermeister, S., & Bunce, D. (2017). A systematic review of longitudinal associations between reaction time intraindividual variability and age-related cognitive decline or impairment, dementia, and mortality. *Journal of the International Neuropsychological Society*, *23*(05), 431–445. https://doi.org/10.1017/S1355617717000236

Hazell, P. L., Kohn, M. R., Dickson, R., Walton, R. J., Granger, R. E., & van Wyk, G. W. (2011). Core ADHD symptom improvement with Atomoxetine versus Methylphenidate: A direct comparison meta-analysis. *Journal of Attention Disorders*, *15*(8), 674–683. https://doi.org/10.1177/1087054710379737

Heathcote, A., Brown, S., & Cousineau, D. (2004). QMPE: Estimating Lognormal, Wald, and Weibull RT distributions with a parameter-dependent lower bound. *Behavior Research Methods, Instruments, and Computers*, *36*(2), 277–290. https://doi.org/10.3758/BF03195574

Heathcote, A., Brown, S., & Mewhort, D. J. K. (2002). Quantile maximum likelihood estimation of response time distributions. *Psychonomic Bulletin and Review*, *9*(2), 394–401. https://doi.org/10.3758/BF03196299

Helps, S. K., Broyd, S. J., Bitsakou, P., & Sonuga-Barke, E. J. S. (2011). Identifying a distinctive familial frequency band in reaction time fluctuations in ADHD. *Neuropsychology*, *25*(6), 711–719. https://doi.org/10.1037/a0024479

Henríquez-Henríquez, M. P., Billeke, P., Henríquez, H., Zamorano, F. J., Rothhammer, F., & Aboitiz, F. (2015). Intra-individual response variability assessed by ex-Gaussian analysis may be a new endophenotype for attention-deficit/hyperactivity disorder. *Frontiers in Psychiatry*, *5*, 1–8. https://doi.org/10.3389/fpsyt.2014.00197

Hervey, A. S., Epstein, J. N., Curry, J. F., Tonev, S., Eugene Arnold, L., Keith Conners, C., … Hechtman, L. (2006). Reaction time distribution analysis of neuropsychological performance in an ADHD sample. *Child Neuropsychology*, *12*(2), 125–140. https://doi.org/10.1080/09297040500499081

Hill, B. D., Rohling, M. L., Boettcher, A. C., & Meyers, J. E. (2013). Cognitive intra-individual variability has a positive association with traumatic brain injury severity and suboptimal effort. *Archives of Clinical Neuropsychology*, *28*(7), 640–648. https://doi.org/10.1093/arclin/act045

Homack, S. R., & Reynolds, C. R. (2007). *Essentials of assessment with brief intelligence tests* (A. S. Kaufman & N. L. Kaufman, Eds.). New Jersey: John Wiley and Sons, Inc.

Hommel, B., Li, K. Z. H., & Li, S.-C. (2004). Visual search across the life span. *Developmental Psychology*, *40*(4), 545–558. https://doi.org/10.1037/0012-1649.40.4.545

Hong, S. B., Zalesky, A., Park, S., Yang, Y. H., Park, M. H., Kim, B., … Kim, J. W. (2015). COMT genotype affects brain white matter pathways in attention-deficit/hyperactivity disorder. *Human Brain Mapping*, *36*(1), 367–377. https://doi.org/10.1002/hbm.22634

Huang-Pollock, C. L., Karalunas, S. L., Tam, H., & Moore, A. N. (2012). Evaluating vigilance deficits in ADHD: A meta-analysis of CPT performance. *Journal of Abnormal Psychology*, *121*(2), 360–371. https://doi.org/10.1037/a0027205

Hultsch, D. F., MacDonald, S. W. S., & Dixon, R. A. (2002). Variability in reaction time performance of younger and older adults. *The Journals of Gerontology. Series B, Psychological Sciences and Social Sciences*, *57*(2), 101–115. Retrieved from http://www.ncbi.nlm.nih.gov/pubmed/11867658

Hultsch, D. F., MacDonald, S. W. S., Hunter, M. A., Levy-Bencheton, J., & Strauss, E. (2000). Intraindividual variability in cognitive performance in older adults: Comparison of adults with mild dementia, adults with arthritis, and healthy adults. *Neuropsychology*, *14*(4), 588–598. https://doi.org/10.1037//0894-4105.14.4.588

Hultsch, D. F., Strauss, E., Hunter, M. A., & MacDonald, S. W. S. (2008). Intraindividual variability, cognition, and aging. In F. I. Craik & T. A. Salthouse (Eds.), *Intraindividual variability, cognition, and aging* (pp. 492–556). New York, NY: Psychology Press.

Hwang-Gu, S. L., Chen, Y. C., Liang, S. H. Y., Ni, H. C., Lin, H. Y., Lin, C. F., & Gau, S. S. F. (2019). Exploring the variability in reaction times of preschoolers at risk of Attention-Deficit/Hyperactivity Disorder: An ex-Gaussian analysis. *Journal of Abnormal Child Psychology*, (7). https://doi.org/10.1007/s10802-018-00508-z

Jackson, J. D., Balota, D. A., Duchek, J. M., & Head, D. (2012). White matter integrity and reaction time intraindividual variability in healthy aging and early-stage Alzheimer disease. *Neuropsychologia*, *50*(3), 357–366. https://doi.org/10.1016/j.neuropsychologia.2011.11.024

Johnson, B. P., Pinar, A., Fornito, A., Nandam, L. S., Hester, R., & Bellgrove, M. A. (2015). Left anterior cingulate activity predicts intra-individual reaction time variability in healthy adults. *Neuropsychologia*, *72*, 22–26. https://doi.org/10.1016/j.neuropsychologia.2015.03.015

Johnson, K. A., Kelly, S. P., Bellgrove, M. A., Barry, E., Cox, M., Gill, M., & Robertson, I. H. (2007). Response variability in Attention Deficit Hyperactivity Disorder: Evidence for neuropsychological heterogeneity. *Neuropsychologia*, *45*(4), 630–638. https://doi.org/10.1016/j.neuropsychologia.2006.03.034

Karalunas, S. L., Geurts, H. M., Konrad, K., Bender, S., & Nigg, J. T. (2014). Annual research review: Reaction time variability in ADHD and autism spectrum disorders: Measurement and mechanisms of a proposed trans-diagnostic phenotype. *Journal of*

Child Psychology and Psychiatry and Allied Disciplines, *55*(6), 685–710. https://doi.org/10.1111/jcpp.12217

Karalunas, S. L., & Huang-Pollock, C. L. (2013). Integrating impairments in reaction time and executive function using a diffusion model framework. *Journal of Abnormal Child Psychology*, *41*(5), 837–850. https://doi.org/10.1007/s10802-013-9715-2

Karalunas, S. L., Huang-Pollock, C. L., & Nigg, J. T. (2013). Is reaction time variability in ADHD mainly at low frequencies? *Journal of Child Psychology and Psychiatry and Allied Disciplines*, *54*(5), 536–544. https://doi.org/10.1111/jcpp.12028

Karalunas, S. L., Nigg, J. T., & Huang-Pollock, C. L. (2012). Decomposing attention-deficit/hyperactivity disorder (ADHD)-related effects in response speed and variability. *Neuropsychology*, *26*(6), 684–694. https://doi.org/10.1037/a0029936

Karr, J. E., Garcia-Barrera, M. A., & Areshenkoff, C. N. (2014). Executive functions and intraindividual variability following concussion. *Journal of Clinical and Experimental Neuropsychology*, *36*(1), 15–31. https://doi.org/10.1080/13803395.2013.863833

Kaufman, A. S., & Kaufman, N. L. (2004). *Kaufman Brief Intelligence Test, Second Edition*. Bloomington, MN: Pearson, Inc.

Kaufman, J., Birmaher, B., Axelson, D., Pereplitchikova, F., Brent, D., & Ryan, N. (2016). KSADS-PL DSM-5. Retrieved from Kennedy Krieger Institute website: https://www.kennedykrieger.org/sites/default/files/library/documents/faculty/ksads-dsm-5-screener.pdf

Kebir, O., & Joober, R. (2011). Neuropsychological endophenotypes in attention-deficit/hyperactivity disorder: A review of genetic association studies. *European Archives of Psychiatry and Clinical Neuroscience*, *261*(8), 583–594. https://doi.org/10.1007/s00406-011-0207-5

Kebir, O., Tabbane, K., Sengupta, S., & Joober, R. (2009). Examen critique Candidate genes and neuropsychological phenotypes in children with ADHD: Review of association studies. *J Psychiatry Neuroscience*, *34*(2), 88–101.

Kelly, A. M. C., Uddin, L. Q., Biswal, B. B., Castellanos, F. X., & Milham, M. P. (2008). Competition between functional brain networks mediates behavioral variability. *NeuroImage*, *39*(1), 527–537. https://doi.org/10.1016/j.neuroimage.2007.08.008

Klein, C., Wendling, K., Huettner, P., Ruder, H., & Peper, M. (2006). *Intra-Subject Variability in Attention-Deficit Hyperactivity Disorder*. https://doi.org/10.1016/j.biopsych.2006.04.003

Klotz, J. M., Johnson, M. D., Wu, S. W., Isaacs, K. M., & Gilbert, D. L. (2012). Relationship between reaction time variability and motor skill development in ADHD. *Child Neuropsychology*, *18*(6), 576–585. https://doi.org/10.1080/09297049.2011.625356

Knopik, V. S., Marceau, K., Bidwell, L. C., Palmer, R. H. C., Smith, T. F., Todorov, A.,

… Heath, A. C. (2016). Smoking during pregnancy and ADHD risk: A genetically informed, multiple-rater approach. *American Journal of Medical Genetics, Part B: Neuropsychiatric Genetics*, *171*(7), 971–981. https://doi.org/10.1002/ajmg.b.32421

Kofler, M. J., Alderson, R. M., Raiker, J. S., Bolden, J., Sarver, D. E., & Rapport, M. D. (2014). Working memory and intraindividual variability as neurocognitive indicators in ADHD: examining competing model predictions. *Neuropsychology*, *28*(3), 459–471. https://doi.org/10.1037/neu0000050

Kofler, M. J., Rapport, M. D., Sarver, D. E., Raiker, J. S., Orban, S. a., Friedman, L. M., & Kolomeyer, E. G. (2013). Reaction time variability in ADHD: A meta-analytic review of 319 studies. *Clinical Psychology Review*, *33*(6), 795–811. https://doi.org/10.1016/j.cpr.2013.06.001

Krain, A. L., & Castellanos, F. X. (2006). Brain development and ADHD. *Clinical Psychology Review*, *26*(4), 433–444. https://doi.org/10.1016/j.cpr.2006.01.005

Kuntsi, J., Eley, T. C., Taylor, A., Hughes, C., Asherson, P., Caspi, A., & Moffitt, T. E. (2004). Co-occurrence of ADHD and low IQ has genetic origins. *American Journal of Medical Genetics*, *124B*(1), 41–47. https://doi.org/10.1002/ajmg.b.20076

Kuntsi, J., & Klein, C. (2011). Intraindividual variability in ADHD and its implications for research of causal links. In *Behavioral neuroscience of attention deficit hyperactivity disorder and its treatment* (pp. 67–91). https://doi.org/10.1007/7854

Kuntsi, J., McLoughlin, G., & Asherson, P. (2006). Attention Deficit Hyperactivity Disorder. *Neuromolecular Medicine*, *8*, 461–484. https://doi.org/10.1385/NMM

Langley, K., Rice, F., Van Den Bree, M. B. M., & Thapar, A. (2005). Maternal smoking during pregnancy as an environmental risk factor for attention deficit hyperactivity disorder. A review. *Minerva Pediatrica*, *57*(6), 359–371.

Lavigne, J. V., Gouze, K. R., Hopkins, J., & Bryant, F. B. (2016). Multi-domain predictors of Attention Deficit/Hyperactivity Disorder symptoms in preschool children: Cross-informant differences. *Child Psychiatry and Human Development*, *47*(6), 841–856. https://doi.org/10.1007/s10578-015-0616-1

Lee, R. W. Y., Jacobson, L. A., Pritchard, A. E., Ryan, M. S., Yu, Q., Denckla, M. B., … Mahone, E. M. (2015). Jitter reduces response-time variability in ADHD: An ex-Gaussian analysis. *Journal of Attention Disorders*, *19*(9), 794–804. https://doi.org/10.1177/1087054712464269

Lee, Y., Yang, H.-J., Chen, V. C., Lee, W.-T., Teng, M.-J., Lin, C.-H., & Gossop, M. (2016). Meta-analysis of quality of life in children and adolescents with ADHD: By both parent proxy-report and child self-report using PedsQL™. *Research in Developmental Disabilities*, *51–52*(110), 160–172. https://doi.org/10.1016/j.ridd.2015.11.009

Lensing, M. B., Zeiner, P., Sandvik, L., & Opjordsmoen, S. (2015). Quality of life in adults aged 50+ with ADHD. *Journal of Attention Disorders*, *19*(5), 405–413. https://doi.org/10.1177/1087054713480035

Leth-Steensen, C., Elbaz, K. Z., & Douglas, V. I. (2000). Mean response times, variability, and skew in the responding of ADHD children: A response time distributional approach. *Acta Psychologica*, *104*(2), 167–190. https://doi.org/10.1016/S0001-6918(00)00019-6

Li, J. J., Cutting, L. E., Ryan, M., Zilioli, M., Denckla, M. B., & Mahone, E. M. (2009). Response variability in rapid automatized naming predicts reading comprehension. *Journal of Clinical and Experimental Neuropsychology*, *31*(7), 877–888. https://doi.org/10.1080/13803390802646973

Li, S. C., Huxhold, O., & Schmiedek, F. (2004). Aging and attenuated processing robustness: Evidence from cognitive and sensorimotor functioning. *Gerontology*, *50*(1), 28–34. https://doi.org/10.1159/000074386

Lin, H. Y., Gau, S. S. F., Huang-Gu, S. L., Shang, C. Y., Wu, Y. H., & Tseng, W. Y. I. (2014). Neural substrates of behavioral variability in attention deficit hyperactivity disorder: Based on ex-Gaussian reaction time distribution and diffusion spectrum imaging tractography. *Psychological Medicine*, *44*(8), 1751–1764. https://doi.org/10.1017/S0033291713001955

Lin, H. Y., Hwang-Gu, S. L., & Gau, S. S. F. (2015). Intra-individual reaction time variability based on ex-Gaussian distribution as a potential endophenotype for attention-deficit/hyperactivity disorder. *Acta Psychiatrica Scandinavica*, *132*(1), 39–50. https://doi.org/10.1111/acps.12393

Liston, C., Cohen, M. M., Teslovich, T., Levenson, D., & Casey, B. J. (2011). Atypical prefrontal connectivity in attention-deficit/hyperactivity disorder: Pathway to disease or pathological end point? *Biological Psychiatry*, *69*(12), 1168–1177. https://doi.org/10.1016/j.biopsych.2011.03.022

MacDonald, S. W. S., Cervenka, S., Farde, L., Nyberg, L., & Bäckman, L. (2009). Extrastriatal dopamine D2 receptor binding modulates intraindividual variability in episodic recognition and executive functioning. *Neuropsychologia*, *47*(11), 2299–2304. https://doi.org/10.1016/j.neuropsychologia.2009.01.016

MacDonald, S. W. S., Li, S.-C., & Bäckman, L. (2009). Neural underpinnings of within-person variability in cognitive functioning. *Psychology and Aging*, *24*(4), 792–808. https://doi.org/10.1037/a0017798

MacDonald, S. W. S., Nyberg, L., & Bäckman, L. (2006). Intra-individual variability in behavior: links to brain structure, neurotransmission and neuronal activity. *Trends in Neurosciences*, *29*(8), 474–480. https://doi.org/10.1016/j.tins.2006.06.011

MacDonald, S. W. S., Nyberg, L., Sandblom, J., Fischer, H., & Bäckman, L. (2008). Increased response-time variability is associated with reduced inferior parietal activation during episodic recognition in aging. *Journal of Cognitive Neuroscience*, *20*, 779–786. https://doi.org/10.1162/jocn.2008.20502

MacDonald, S. W. S., & Stawski, R. S. (2015). Intraindividual variability- An indicator of vulnerability or resilience in adult development and aging? In M. Diehl, K. Hooker, & M. J. Sliwinski (Eds.), *Handbook of intraindividual variability across the life span* (pp. 231–257). New York, NY: Routlledge Taylor & Francis group.

Maguire, S. A., Williams, B., Naughton, A. M., Cowley, L. E., Tempest, V., Mann, M. K., … Kemp, A. M. (2015). A systematic review of the emotional, behavioural and cognitive features exhibited by school-aged children experiencing neglect or emotional abuse. *Child: Care, Health and Development, 41*(5), 641–653. https://doi.org/10.1111/cch.12227

Mahone, E. M., Ranta, M. E., Crocetti, D., O'Brien, J., Kaufmann, W. E., Denckla, M. B., & Mostofsky, S. H. (2011). Comprehensive examination of frontal regions in boys and girls with attention-deficit/hyperactivity disorder. *Journal of the International Neuropsychological Society, 17*(6), 1047–1057. https://doi.org/10.1017/S1355617711001056

Marcos-Vidal, L., Martínez-García, M., Pretus, C., Garcia-Garcia, D., Martínez, K., Janssen, J., … Carmona, S. (2018). Local functional connectivity suggests functional immaturity in children with attention-deficit/hyperactivity disorder. *Human Brain Mapping, 39*(6), 2442–2454. https://doi.org/10.1002/hbm.24013

McIntosh, A. R., Kovacevic, N., & Itier, R. J. (2008). Increased brain signal variability accompanies lower behavioral variability in development. *PLoS Computational Biology, 4*(7), e1000106. https://doi.org/10.1371/journal.pcbi.1000106

McLoughlin, G., Palmer, J. A., Rijsdijk, F., & Makeig, S. (2014). Genetic overlap between evoked frontocentral theta-band phase variability, reaction time variability, and attention-deficit/hyperactivity disorder symptoms in a twin study. *Biological Psychiatry, 75*(3), 238–247. https://doi.org/10.1016/j.biopsych.2013.07.020

Moy, G., Millet, P., Haller, S., Baudois, S., de Bilbao, F., Weber, K., … Delaloye, C. (2011). Magnetic resonance imaging determinants of intraindividual variability in the elderly: Combined analysis of grey and white matter. *Neuroscience, 186*, 88–93. https://doi.org/10.1016/j.neuroscience.2011.04.028

Muñoz-Silva, A., Lago-Urbano, R., & Sanchez-Garcia, M. (2017). Family impact and parenting styles in families of children with ADHD. *Journal of Child and Family Studies, 26*(10), 2810–2823. https://doi.org/10.1007/s10826-017-0798-1

Murtha, S., Cismaru, R., Waechter, R., & Chertkow, H. (2002). Increased variability accompanies frontal lobe damage in dementia. *Journal of the International Neuropsychological Society, 8*(3), 360–372. https://doi.org/10.1017/S1355617702813170

Naglieri, J. A., & Goldstein, S. (2013). *Comprehensive Executive Function Inventory: Manual.* Multi-Health Systems.

Narad, M. E., Garner, A. A., Peugh, J. L., Tamm, L., Antonini, T. N., Kingery, K. M., … Epstein, J. N. (2015). Parent-teacher agreement on ADHD symptoms across development. *Psychological Assessment, 27*(1), 239–248. https://doi.org/10.1037/a0037864

Nesselroade, J. R. (1991). The warp and the woof of the developmental fabric. In R. M.

Downs, L. S. Liben, & D. S. Palermo (Eds.), *Visions of aesthetics, the environment, and development: The legacy of Joachim F. Wohlwill* (pp. 213–240). Hillsdale, NJ: Lawrence Erlbaum Associates, Inc.

Ni, H.-C., Gu, S.-L. H., Lin, H.-Y., Lin, Y.-J., Yang, L.-K., Huang, H.-C., & Gau, S. S.-F. (2016). Atomoxetine could improve intra-individual variability in drug-naive adults with attention-deficit/hyperactivity disorder comparably with methylphenidate: A head-to-head randomized clinical trial. *Journal of Psychopharmacology*, *30*(5), 459–467. https://doi.org/10.1177/0269881116632377

Nigg, J. T. (2010). Attention-Deficit/Hyperactivity Disorder. *Current Directions in Psychological Science*, *19*(1), 24–29. https://doi.org/10.1177/0963721409359282

Nigg, J. T., Blaskey, L. G., Stawicki, J. A., & Sachek, J. (2004). Evaluating the endophenotype model of ADHD neuropsychological deficit: Results for parents and siblings of children with ADHD combined and inattentive subtypes. *Journal of Abnormal Psychology*, *113*(4), 614–625. https://doi.org/10.1037/0021-843X.113.4.614

Nigg, J. T., Lewis, K., Edinger, T., & Falk, M. (2012). Meta-analysis of attention-deficit/hyperactivity disorder or attention-deficit/hyperactivity disorder symptoms, restriction diet, and synthetic food color additives. *Journal of the American Academy of Child and Adolescent Psychiatry*, *51*(1), 86–97. https://doi.org/10.1016/j.jaac.2011.10.015

Nigg, J. T., Nikolas, M., Knottnerus, M. G., Cavanagh, K., & Friderici, K. (2010). Confirmation and extension of association of blood lead with attention-deficit/hyperactivity disorder (ADHD) and ADHD symptom domains at population-typical exposure levels. *Journal of Child Psychology and Psychiatry and Allied Disciplines*, *51*(1), 58–65. https://doi.org/10.1111/j.1469-7610.2009.02135.x

Parens, E., & Johnston, J. (2009). Facts, values, and attention-deficit hyperactivity disorder (ADHD): An update on the controversies. *Child and Adolescent Psychiatry and Mental Health*, *3*(1), 1. https://doi.org/10.1186/1753-2000-3-1

Pelsser, L. M., Frankena, K., Toorman, J., & Pereira, R. R. (2017). Diet and ADHD, reviewing the evidence: A systematic review of meta-analyses of double-blind placebo-controlled trials evaluating the efficacy of diet interventions on the behavior of children with ADHD. *PLoS ONE*, *12*(1). https://doi.org/10.1371/journal.pone.0169277

Pereira, P. P. D. S., Da Mata, F. A. F., Figueiredo, A. C. G., de Andrade, K. R. C., & Pereira, M. G. (2017). Maternal active smoking during pregnancy and low birth weight in the americas: A systematic review and meta-analysis. *Nicotine and Tobacco Research*, *19*(5), 497–505. https://doi.org/10.1093/ntr/ntw228

Pinto, R., Asherson, P., Ilott, N., Cheung, C. H. M., & Kuntsi, J. (2016). Testing for the mediating role of endophenotypes using molecular genetic data in a twin study of ADHD traits. *American Journal of Medical Genetics, Part B: Neuropsychiatric Genetics*, *171*(7), 982–992. https://doi.org/10.1002/ajmg.b.32463

Ramchurn, A., de Fockert, J. W., Mason, L., Darling, S., & Bunce, D. (2014). Intraindividual reaction time variability affects P300 amplitude rather than latency. *Frontiers in Human Neuroscience*, *8*, 557–565. https://doi.org/10.3389/fnhum.2014.00557

Renart, A., & Machens, C. K. (2014). Variability in neural activity and behavior. *Current Opinion in Neurobiology*, *25*, 211–220. https://doi.org/10.1016/j.conb.2014.02.013

Rossi, A. S. U., de Moura, L. M., de Mello, C. B., de Souza, A. A. L., Muszkat, M., & Bueno, O. F. A. (2015). Attentional profiles and white matter correlates in attention-deficit/hyperactivity disorder predominantly inattentive type. *Frontiers in Psychiatry*, *6*, 122–131. https://doi.org/10.3389/fpsyt.2015.00122

Rowland, A. S., Skipper, B. J., Rabiner, D. L., Qeadan, F., Campbell, R. A., Naftel, A. J., & Umbach, D. M. (2017). Attention-Deficit/Hyperactivity Disorder (ADHD): Interaction between socioeconomic status and parental history of ADHD determines prevalence. *Journal of Child Psychology and Psychiatry*, *59*(3), 213–222. https://doi.org/10.1111/jcpp.12775

Rubia, K. (2011). "Cool" inferior frontostriatal dysfunction in attention-deficit/hyperactivity disorder versus "hot" ventromedial orbitofrontal-limbic dysfunction in conduct disorder: A review. *Biological Psychiatry*, *69*(12), e69–e87. https://doi.org/10.1016/j.biopsych.2010.09.023

Rubia, K., Halari, R., Cubillo, A., Smith, A. B., Mohammad, A. M., Brammer, M., & Taylor, E. (2011). Methylphenidate normalizes fronto-striatal underactivation during interference inhibition in medication-nave boys with attention-deficit hyperactivity disorder. *Neuropsychopharmacology*, *36*(8), 1575–1586. https://doi.org/10.1038/npp.2011.30

Rubia, K., Smith, A. B., Brammer, M. J., & Taylor, E. (2007). Temporal lobe dysfunction in medication-naïve boys with Attention-Deficit/Hyperactivity Disorder during attention allocation and its relation to response variability. *Biological Psychiatry*, *62*(9), 999–1006. https://doi.org/10.1016/j.biopsych.2007.02.024

Russell, A. E., Ford, T., Williams, R., & Russell, G. (2016). The association between socioeconomic disadvantage and Attention Deficit/Hyperactivity Disorder (ADHD): A systematic review. *Child Psychiatry and Human Development*, *47*(3), 440–458. https://doi.org/10.1007/s10578-015-0578-3

Russell, V. A., Oades, R. D., Tannock, R., Killeen, P. R., Auerbach, J. G., Johansen, E. B., & Sagvolden, T. (2006). Response variability in Attention-Deficit/Hyperactivity Disorder: A neuronal and glial energetics hypothesis. *Behavioral and Brain Functions*, *2*(1), 30. https://doi.org/10.1186/1744-9081-2-30

Ryan, M., Jacobson, L. A., Hague, C., Bellows, A., Denckla, M. B., & Mahone, E. M. (2017). Rapid automatized naming (RAN) in children with ADHD: An ex-Gaussian analysis. *Child Neuropsychology*, *23*(5), 571–587. https://doi.org/10.1080/09297049.2016.1172560

Saville, C. W. N., Feige, B., Kluckert, C., Bender, S., Biscaldi, M., Berger, A., … Klein,

C. (2015). Increased reaction time variability in attention-deficit hyperactivity disorder as a response-related phenomenon: Evidence from single-trial event-related potentials. *Journal of Child Psychology and Psychiatry and Allied Disciplines*, *56*(7), 801–813. https://doi.org/10.1111/jcpp.12348

Schei, J., Jozefiak, T., Nøvik, T. S., Lydersen, S., & Indredavik, M. S. (2016). The impact of coexisting emotional and conduct problems on family functioning and quality of life among adolescents with ADHD. *Journal of Attention Disorders*, *20*(5), 424–433. https://doi.org/10.1177/1087054713507976

Schmiedek, F., Oberauer, K., Wilhelm, O., Süß, H.-M., & Wittmann, W. W. (2007). Individual differences in components of reaction time distributions and their relations to working memory and intelligence. *Journal of Experimental Psychology: General*, *136*(3), 414–429. https://doi.org/10.1037/0096-3445.136.3.414

Schneider, M. F., Krick, C. M., Retz, W., Hengesch, G., Retz-Junginger, P., Reith, W., & Rösler, M. (2010). Impairment of fronto-striatal and parietal cerebral networks correlates with attention deficit hyperactivity disorder (ADHD) psychopathology in adults - A functional magnetic resonance imaging (fMRI) study. *Psychiatry Research - Neuroimaging*, *183*(1), 75–84. https://doi.org/10.1016/j.pscychresns.2010.04.005

Schweren, L. J. S., Hartman, C. A., Zwiers, M. P., Heslenfeld, D. J., Franke, B., Oosterlaan, J., … Hoekstra, P. J. (2016). Stimulant treatment history predicts frontal-striatal structural connectivity in adolescents with attention-deficit/hyperactivity disorder. *European Neuropsychopharmacology*, *26*(4), 674–683. https://doi.org/10.1016/j.euroneuro.2016.02.007

Sergeant, J. A. (2005). Modeling attention-deficit/hyperactivity disorder: A critical appraisal of the cognitive-energetic model. *Biological Psychiatry*, *57*(11), 1248–1255. https://doi.org/10.1016/j.biopsych.2004.09.010

Shaw, R., Grayson, A., & Lewis, V. (2005). Inhibition, ADHD, and computer games : ADHD on computerized tasks and games. *Journal of Attention Disorders*, *8*(4), 160–168. https://doi.org/10.1177/1087054705278771

Silva, D., Colvin, L., Hagemann, E., & Bower, C. (2014). Environmental risk factors by gender associated with Attention-Deficit/Hyperactivity Disorder. *Pediatrics*, *133*(1), e14–e22. https://doi.org/10.1542/peds.2013-1434

Simmonds, D. J., Fotedar, S. G., Suskauer, S. J., Pekar, J. J., Denckla, M. B., & Mostofsky, S. H. (2007). Functional brain correlates of response time variability in children. *Neuropsychologia*, *45*(9), 2147–2157. https://doi.org/10.1016/j.neuropsychologia.2007.01.013

Sims, D. M., & Lonigan, C. J. (2012). Multi-method assessment of ADHD characteristics in preschool children: Relations between measures. *Early Childhood Research Quarterly*, *27*(2), 329–337. https://doi.org/10.1016/j.ecresq.2011.08.004

Sinclair, K. L., Ponsford, J. L., Rajaratnam, S. M. W., & Anderson, C. (2013). Sustained attention following traumatic brain injury: Use of the Psychomotor Vigilance Task.

Journal of Clinical and Experimental Neuropsychology, *35*(2), 210–224. https://doi.org/10.1080/13803395.2012.762340

Sliwinski, M. J., Smyth, J. M., Hofer, S. M., & Stawski, R. S. (2006). Intraindividual coupling of daily stress and cognition. *Psychology and Aging*, *21*(3), 545–557. https://doi.org/10.1037/0882-7974.21.3.545

Sonuga-Barke, E. J. S., Brandeis, D., Cortese, S., Daley, D., Ferrin, M., Holtmann, M., … Zuddas, A. (2013). Nonpharmacological interventions for ADHD: Systematic review and meta-analyses of randomized controlled trials of dietary and psychological treatments. *American Journal of Psychiatry*, *170*(3), 275–289. https://doi.org/10.1176/appi.ajp.2012.12070991

Sonuga-Barke, E. J. S., & Castellanos, F. X. (2007). Spontaneous attentional fluctuations in impaired states and pathological conditions: A neurobiological hypothesis. *Neuroscience and Biobehavioral Reviews*, *31*(7), 977–986. https://doi.org/10.1016/j.neubiorev.2007.02.005

Sonuga-Barke, E. J. S., & Halperin, J. M. (2010). Developmental phenotypes and causal pathways in attention deficithyperactivity disorder: Potential targets for early intervention? *Journal of Child Psychology and Psychiatry and Allied Disciplines*, *51*(4), 368–389. https://doi.org/10.1111/j.1469-7610.2009.02195.x

Sonuga-Barke, E. J. S., Koerting, J., Smith, E., McCann, D. C., & Thompson, M. (2011). Early detection and intervention for attention-deficit/hyperactivity disorder. *Expert Review of Neurotherapeutics*, *11*(4), 557–563.

Sosnoff, J. J., Broglio, S. P., Hillman, C. H., & Ferrara, M. S. (2007). Concussion does not impact intraindividual response time variability. *Neuropsychology*, *21*(6), 796–802. https://doi.org/10.1037/0894-4105.21.6.796

Spencer, S. V., Hawk, L. W., Richards, J. B., Shiels, K., Pelham, W. E., & Waxmonsky, J. G. (2009). Stimulant treatment reduces lapses in attention among children with ADHD: The effects of methylphenidate on intra-individual response time distributions. *Journal of Abnormal Child Psychology*, *37*(6), 805–816. https://doi.org/10.1007/s10802-009-9316-2

Stawski, R. S., MacDonald, S. W. S., Brewster, P. W. H., Munoz, E., Cerino, E. S., & Halliday, D. W. R. (2019). A comprehensive comparison of quantifications of intraindividual variability in response times: A measurement burst approach. *The Journals of Gerontology: Series B*, *74*(3), 397–408. https://doi.org/10.1093/geronb/gbx115

Stukas, A. A., & Cumming, G. (2014). Special issue article : Methods and statistics in social psychology : Re fi nements and new developments Exploring social and personal relationships : The issue of measurement invariance of non-independent observations. *European Journal of Social Psychology*, *690*(May), 683–690. https://doi.org/10.1002/ejsp.2042

Stuss, D. T., Murphy, K. J., Binns, M. A., & Alexander, M. P. (2003). Staying on the job: the frontal lobes control individual performance variability. *Brain : A Journal of*

Neurology, *126*(11), 2363–2380. https://doi.org/10.1093/brain/awg237

Suskauer, S. J., Simmonds, D. J., Caffo, B. S., Denckla, M. B., Pekar, J. J., & Mostofsky, S. H. (2008). fMRI of intrasubject variability in ADHD: anomalous premotor activity with prefrontal compensation. *Journal of the American Academy of Child and Adolescent Psychiatry*, *47*(10), 1141–1150. https://doi.org/10.1097/CHI.0b013e3181825b1f

Tallberg, P., Råstam, M., Wenhov, L., Eliasson, G., & Gustafsson, P. (2019). Incremental clinical utility of continuous performance tests in childhood ADHD – an evidence-based assessment approach. *Scandinavian Journal of Psychology*, *60*(1), 26–35. https://doi.org/10.1111/sjop.12499

Tamm, L., Epstein, J. N., Denton, C. A., Vaughn, A. J., Peugh, J., & Willcutt, E. G. (2014). Reaction Time Variability Associated with Reading Skills in Poor Readers with ADHD. *Journal of the International Neuropsychological Society*, *20*(03), 292–301. https://doi.org/10.1017/S1355617713001495

Tamm, L., Narad, M. E., Antonini, T. N., O'Brien, K. M., Hawk, L. W., & Epstein, J. N. (2012). Reaction time variability in ADHD: A review. *Neurotherapeutics*, *9*(3), 500–508. https://doi.org/10.1007/s13311-012-0138-5

Tamnes, C. K., Fjell, A. M., Westlye, L. T., Ostby, Y., & Walhovd, K. B. (2012). Becoming consistent: Developmental reductions in intraindividual variability in reaction time are related to white matter integrity. *Journal of Neuroscience*, *32*(3), 972–982. https://doi.org/10.1523/JNEUROSCI.4779-11.2012

Tang, H., Huang, J., Nie, K., Gan, R., Wang, L., Zhao, J., … Wang, L. (2016). Cognitive profile of Parkinson's disease patients: A comparative study between early-onset and late-onset Parkinson's disease. *International Journal of Neuroscience*, *126*(3), 227–234. https://doi.org/10.3109/00207454.2015.1010646

Tarantino, V., Cutini, S., Mogentale, C., & Bisiacchi, P. S. (2013). Time-on-task in children with ADHD: An ex-Gaussian analysis. *Journal of the International Neuropsychological Society*, *19*(7), 820–828. https://doi.org/10.1017/S1355617713000623

Tarver, J., Daley, D., & Sayal, K. (2014). Attention-deficit hyperactivity disorder (ADHD): An updated review of the essential facts. *Child: Care, Health and Development*, *40*(6), 762–774. https://doi.org/10.1111/cch.12139

Thapar, A., & Cooper, M. (2016). Attention deficit hyperactivity disorder. *The Lancet*, *387*, 1240–1250. https://doi.org/10.1016/S0140-6736(15)00238-X

Thapar, A., Cooper, M., Eyre, O., & Langley, K. (2013). Practitioner review: What have we learnt about the causes of ADHD? *Journal of Child Psychology and Psychiatry and Allied Disciplines*, *54*(1), 3–16. https://doi.org/10.1111/j.1469-7610.2012.02611.x

Thissen, A. J. A. M., Luman, M., Hartman, C., Hoekstra, P., Van Lieshout, M., Franke, B., … Buitelaar, J. K. (2014). Attention-Deficit/Hyperactivity Disorder (ADHD)

and motor timing in adolescents and their parents: Familial characteristics of reaction time variability vary with age. *Journal of the American Academy of Child and Adolescent Psychiatry*, *53*(9), 1010–1019. https://doi.org/10.1016/j.jaac.2014.05.015

Tripp, G., Luk, S. L., Schaughency, E. A., & Singh, R. (1999). DSM-IV and ICD-10: A comparison of the correlates of ADHD and hyperkinetic disorder. *Journal of the American Academy of Child and Adolescent Psychiatry*, *38*(2), 156–164. https://doi.org/10.1097/00004583-199902000-00014

Tye, C., Johnson, K. A., Kelly, S. P., Asherson, P., Kuntsi, J., Ashwood, K. L., … McLoughlin, G. (2016). Response time variability under slow and fast-incentive conditions in children with ASD, ADHD and ASD+ADHD. *Journal of Child Psychology and Psychiatry and Allied Disciplines*, *57*(12), 1414–1423. https://doi.org/10.1111/jcpp.12608

Uebel, H., Albrecht, B., Asherson, P., Börger, N. A., Butler, L., Chen, W., … Banaschewski, T. (2010). Performance variability, impulsivity errors and the impact of incentives as gender-independent endophenotypes for ADHD. *Journal of Child Psychology and Psychiatry and Allied Disciplines*, *51*(2), 210–218. https://doi.org/10.1111/j.1469-7610.2009.02139.x

van Ewijk, H., Heslenfeld, D. J., Zwiers, M. P., Buitelaar, J. K., & Oosterlaan, J. (2012). Diffusion tensor imaging in attention deficit/hyperactivity disorder: A systematic review and meta-analysis. *Neuroscience and Biobehavioral Reviews*, *36*(4), 1093–1106. https://doi.org/10.1016/j.neubiorev.2012.01.003

Vaughan, B. S., March, J. S., & Kratochvil, C. J. (2012). The evidence-based pharmacological treatment of paediatric ADHD. *The International Journal of Neuropsychopharmacology / Official Scientific Journal of the Collegium Internationale Neuropsychopharmacologicum (CINP)*, *15*(1), 27–39. https://doi.org/10.1017/S1461145711000095

Vaurio, R. G., Simmonds, D. J., & Mostofsky, S. H. (2009). Increased intra-individual reaction time variability in attention- deficit/hyperactivity disorder across response inhibition tasks with different cognitive demands. *Neuropsychologia*, *47*(12), 2389–2396. https://doi.org/10.1146/annurev-immunol-032713-120240.Microglia

Wagenmakers, E.-J., & Brown, S. (2007). On the linear relation between the mean and the standard deviation of a response time distribution. *Psychological Review*, *114*(3), 830–841. https://doi.org/10.1037/0033-295X.114.3.830

Walhovd, K. B., & Fjell, A. M. (2007). White matter volume predicts reaction time instability. *Neuropsychologia*, *45*(10), 2277–2284. https://doi.org/10.1016/j.neuropsychologia.2007.02.022

Weissman, D. H., Roberts, K. C., Visscher, K. M., & Woldorff, M. G. (2006). The neural bases of momentary lapses in attention. *Nature Neuroscience*, *9*(7), 971–978. https://doi.org/10.1038/nn1727

WHO. (2004). *The ICD-10: International statistical classification of diseases and related health problems: Tenth revision* (2nd ed.). Geneva: World Health Oganization.

Williams, B. R., Hultsch, D. F., Strauss, E. H., Hunter, M. A., & Tannock, R. (2005). Inconsistency in reaction time across the life span. *Neuropsychology*, *19*(1), 88–96. https://doi.org/10.1037/0894-4105.19.1.88

Wolfers, T., Onnink, A. M. H., Zwiers, M. P., Arias-Vasquez, A., Hoogman, M., Mostert, J. C., … Franke, B. (2015). Lower white matter microstructure in the superior longitudinal fasciculus is associated with increased response time variability in adults with attentiondeficit/hyperactivity disorder. *Journal of Psychiatry and Neuroscience*, *40*(5), 344–351. https://doi.org/10.1503/jpn.140154

Zakzanis, K. K. (2001). Statistics to tell the truth, the whole truth, and nothing but the truth. Formulae, illustrative numerical examples, and heuristic interpretation of effect size analyses for neuropsychological researchers. *Archives of Clinical Neuropsychology*, *16*(7), 653–667. https://doi.org/10.1016/S0887-6177(00)00076-7

Zimmermann, P., Gondan, M., & Fimm, B. (2005). *Test of Attention Performance for Children*. Herzogenrath: Psytest.

Appendix A

Participant Screening Questions

1) Is your child a boy or girl?
2) How old is your child ***(must be 6-13 to be include in study)***
3) What grade is your child in?
4) Does your child have a formal diagnosis of Attention Deficit Hyperactivity Disorder?

If Yes:

a. When was this diagnosis made? (date, grade, or approximate age of child OK, age best)
b. Who made this diagnosis? (psychiatrist, psychologist, GP, pediatrician, other)
c. Was your child given the diagnosis of ADHD predominantly inattentive, predominantly hyperactive/impulsive, or combined presentation?
d. Does your child take medications to manage ADHD?
If yes, Which ADHD medications does your child take?
e. How long has your child taken this medication for?

5) Does your child take any (other) medications?

6) Does your child hold any other specific diagnoses, such as a:

a. Learning Disability, ***(Yes*/No)** **(Yes ok for ADHD only)**
b. Oppositional Defiant Disorder **(Yes/No) (Yes ok for ADHD only)**
c. Intellectual disability, **(Yes/No)**
d. Autism Spectrum Disorder? **(Yes/No)**
e. other neurodevelopmental disorders (e.g., Fetal Alcohol Spectrum Disorder)? **(Yes/No)**

(for study participation in <u>ADHD group</u>, it is OK if they have comorbid Learning Disability or Oppositional Defiant Disorder, but not if they have an Intellectual Disability or Autism or other neurodevelopmental disorder (FASD, etc.); for control group must be no to all.)

7) Does your child have any diagnosed medical conditions?

8) Does your child have any diagnosed mental health conditions (e.g., anxiety, depression, etc.)?

(for both groups OK if the child has experienced some anxiety or depression, but not for a child who is currently severely anxious or depressed i.e. diagnosed and/or taking medications for this. Participants with bipolar disorder or childhood schizophrenia would not be eligible).

Appendix B

CHILD HISTORY SCREENING QUESTIONNAIRE

This questionnaire was designed as a measure to obtain basic information about your child. Whatever information you may be able to offer will be invaluable in helping us to determine which applicants are most suitable for this phase of the study. We appreciate your participation in what we feel is an exciting and important study.

Child's name ______________________________ Sex M _____ F _____

Date of Birth ______________________________ Age ____________________

Parent(s) Name__________________ Phone No.______________
Email.________________

Postal Code __________________

Annual Income (*entire home; Check one)*

- ○ 0-40,000
- ○ 40,001 – 75,000
- ○ 75,001 - 90,000
- ○ 90,001 - 100,000
- ○ Over 100,000

Ethnicity _________________
First language ______________

DEVELOPMENTAL/MEDICAL HISTORY

Pregnancy with this child:

Were there any complications with your pregnancy with this child (e.g. anemia, high blood pressure, toxemia, diabetes, infections, hospitalizations, etc.). (If yes, please specify)

____

____

Were any medications/drugs used during the pregnancy (If yes, please specify)

____

____

Complications during birth:

Induced ______

C-Section ______

Forceps ______

Fetal Distress ______

Breech (feet First) ______

Twins ______

Other (e.g. breathing problems, cord around neck):______________________________

Newborn:

Following delivery, was the baby:

Blue at birth ______

Require oxygen ______

Have jaundice ______

Require Phototherapy.

Have seizures ______

Other: ______________________________

Was medication used? Yes ________ No ________ If yes, reason.
____

Childhood:

Has your child ever experienced:

Very high fever	______	Polio	______	Dizzy spells
Measles	______	Whooping Cough	______	Frequent colds
Mumps	______	Chicken Pox	______	Scarlet Fever
Seizures	______	Asthma	______	Freq. Ear infections
Meningitis	______	Encephalitis	______	Head injuries
Heart Disease	______	Migraines	______	Headaches
AIDS	______	Visual defects	______	Hearing defects

Other: ______________________________

Food Allergies: ______________________________

Drug Allergies: ______________________________

Did your child have any early developmental problems, such as delayed walking or talking or other. If yes, please specify
____
____

Are there any medical problems currently affecting your child. If yes, please explain.
____
____

Is your child currently taking medication (specify specific medication and dosage)?
____
____

Does your child have any psychological/mental health or psychiatric diagnoses? (e.g., ADHD, Learning Disability, anxiety/depression, etc.). If yes, please specify:

1. Specific diagnosis/diagnoses:

____

____

2. Date of diagnosis/diagnoses:

____

____

3. Diagnosis/diagnoses made by which type of professional (circle which one(s) applies)

a. pediatrician b. psychiatrist c. family physician/GP

b. counsellor d. other (please specify):________________

Has your child received or been involved in any of the following services of supports?

	Grade/Age
Learning Disabilities/Special Education Class	______
Behavioral Adjustment Class	______
Tutoring	______
Enrichment/Gifted	______
Language Immersion	______
Counselling	______
Speech Language Services	______
Occupational Therapy Services	______
Social Skills/Friendship Groups	______
Mental health Counselling	______

Other (please specify): _______________________________

Appendix C

DSM-5 Diagnostic Criteria for Attention Deficit/Hyperactivity Disorder

A. A persistent pattern of inattention and/or hyperactivity-impulsivity that interferes with functioning or development, as characterized by (1) and/or (2):
   1. Inattention: Six (or more) of the following symptoms have persisted for at least 6 months to a degree that is inconsistent with developmental level and that negatively impacts directly on social and academic/occupational activities: Note: The symptoms are not solely a manifestation of oppositional behavior, defiance, hostility, or failure to understand tasks or instructions. For older adolescents and adults (age 17 and older), at least five symptoms are required.
      a. Often fails to give close attention to details or makes careless mistakes in schoolwork, at work, or during other activities (e.g., overlooks or misses details, work is inaccurate).
      b. Often has difficulty sustaining attention in tasks or play activities (e.g., has difficulty remaining focused during lectures, conversations, or lengthy reading).
      c. Often does not seem to listen when spoken to directly (e.g., mind seems elsewhere, even in the absence of any obvious distraction).
      d. Often does not follow through on instructions and fails to finish schoolwork, chores, or duties in the workplace (e.g., starts tasks but quickly loses focus and is easily sidetracked).
      e. Often has difficulty organizing tasks and activities (e.g., difficulty managing sequential tasks; difficulty keeping materials and belongings in order; messy, disorganized work; has poor time management; fails to meet deadlines).
      f. Often avoids, dislikes, or is reluctant to engage in tasks that require sustained mental effort (e.g., schoolwork or homework; for older adolescents and adults, preparing reports, completing forms, reviewing lengthy papers).
      g. Often loses things necessary for tasks or activities (e.g., school materials, pencils, books, tools, wallets, keys, paperwork, eyeglasses, mobile telephones).
      h. Is often easily distracted by extraneous stimuli (for older adolescents and adults, may include unrelated thoughts).
      i. Is often forgetful in daily activities (e.g., doing chores, running errands; for older adolescents and adults, returning calls, paying bills, keeping appointments).

2. Hyperactivity and impulsivity: Six (or more) of the following symptoms have persisted for at least 6 months to a degree that is inconsistent with developmental level and that negatively impacts directly on social and academic/occupational activities: Note: The symptoms are not solely a manifestation of oppositional behavior, defiance, hostility, or a failure to understand tasks or instructions. For older adolescents and adults (age 17 and older), at least five symptoms are required.
    a. Often fidgets with or taps hands or feet or squirms in seat.
    b. Often leaves seat in situations when remaining seated is expected (e.g., leaves his or her place in the classroom, in the office or other workplace, or in other situations that require remaining in place).
    c. Often runs about or climbs in situations where it is inappropriate. (Note: In adolescents or adults, may be limited to feeling restless.)
    d. Often unable to play or engage in leisure activities quietly.
    e. Is often "on the go," acting as if "driven by a motor" (e.g., is unable to be or uncomfortable being still for extended time, as in restaurants, meetings; may be experienced by others as being restless or difficult to keep up with).
    f. Often talks excessively.
    g. Often blurts out an answer before a question has been completed (e.g., completes people's sentences; cannot wait for turn in conversation).
    h. Often has difficulty waiting his or her turn (e.g., while waiting in line).
    i. Often interrupts or intrudes on others (e.g., butts into conversations, games, or activities; may start using other people's things without asking or receiving permission; for adolescents and adults, may intrude into or take over what others are doing).

B. Several inattentive or hyperactive-impulsive symptoms were present prior to age 12 years.

C. Several inattentive or hyperactive-impulsive symptoms are present in two or more settings (e.g., at home, school, or work; with friends or relatives; in other activities).

D. There is clear evidence that the symptoms interfere with, or reduce the quality of, social, academic, or occupational functioning.

E. The symptoms do not occur exclusively during the course of schizophrenia or another psychotic disorder and are not better explained by another mental disorder (e.g., mood disorder, anxiety disorder, dissociative disorder, personality disorder, substance intoxication or withdrawal).

Specify whether:

314.01 (F90.2) **Combined presentation**: If both Criterion A1 (inattention) and Criterion A2 (hyperactivity-impulsivity) are met for the past 6 months.
314.00 (F90.0) **Predominantly inattentive presentation**: If Criterion A1 (inattention) is met but Criterion A2 (hyperactivity-impulsivity) is not met for the past 6 months.
314.01 (F90.1) **Predominantly hyperactive/impulsive presentation**: If Criterion A2 (hyperactivityimpulsivity) is met but Criterion A1 (inattention) is not met over the past 6 months.

Specify if:

In partial remission: When full criteria were previously met, fewer than the full criteria have been met for the past 6 months, and the symptoms still result in impairment in social, academic, or occupational functioning.

Specify current severity:

Mild: Few, if any, symptoms in excess of those required to make the diagnosis are present, and symptoms result in only minor functional impairments.
Moderate: Symptoms or functional impairment between "mild" and "severe" are present.
Severe: Many symptoms in excess of those required to make the diagnosis, or several symptoms that are particularly severe, are present, or the symptoms result in marked impairment in social or occupational functioning.

www.ingramcontent.com/pod-product-compliance
Lightning Source LLC
LaVergne TN
LVHW041117150826
845673LV00007B/2100

* 9 7 8 3 3 8 4 2 2 2 0 5 3 *